# Intestinal Parasites
## AND THE
# Meaning of Life

Written & Illustrated by Scott W. Webb

# CONTENTS

"This means war!"

Groucho Marx

# Introduction

By way of a heads up, what's presented here will be generally regarded as <u>outrageous</u>. I know that! It's outrageous to <u>me</u>.

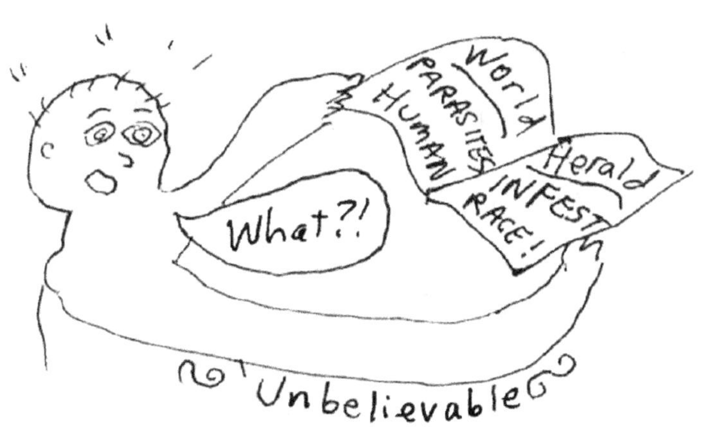

So rather than putting your thinking cap on, I'm going to ask that you take it off.

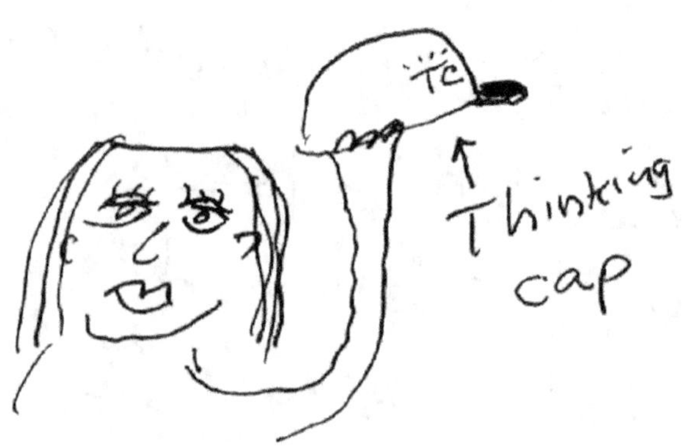


Because what you are going to explore here will defy logic and the way we categorize things in our brains.

I didn't choose this topic. The topic chose me. I understand that most people know very little about their internal organs and many would be challenged to merely point to where their liver is located in their own body or to trace the shape of their colon. That's okay! But it's _time to get serious_.

I know that people don't want to think about their poop because the common paradigm is what <u>matters</u> is what one puts <u>into</u> their mouth and there it stops.



Below here:
<u>No</u> man's <u>land</u>

The majority of this book will stand in contrast to what doctors believe, including nurses, lab technicians, scientists, hospital administrators, clinic specialists and <u>their janitors</u> too. But it's also more than that, because others who would put their foot down and say NO to it include chiropractors, acupuncturists, psychiatrists, aromatherapists, Ayurvedic experts, energy healers, naturopaths, yoga instructors,

and even many colon
hygienists shy away
from emphasizing human
parasites, which is how
I was about it, until
recently.  Something for
me changed, which I'll
cover, how that came about.
later
        I've been particularly
blessed in the health
department. I've had zero
illnesses for the past 20
years and none to speak
of before that.  ~~Bu~~ My
parents gave my new bride
and me a juicer as a
        wedding gift →

back in 1984 and we used it, almost daily, and I still juice almost daily, some days fruits, other days vegetables, including greens such as parsley. I've had a garden for the past seven or eight years, prefer organically grown food, make my own ferments, use miso in my diet, exercise regularly, you get the idea.

One major difference about me is that I notice <u>little</u> <u>differences</u>.

For example, a friend of mine's husband passed away a few years ago in his forties and the last time I had seen him before that, he was a strapping picture of <u>vitality</u>. My friend recounted that in his final months, he suffered from a terrible <u>itching</u>, then died. Now I am not a hypochondriac, but about a year ago, I noticed that my body was itching.

It was when I stepped
into the shower, and
mostly along one side of
my back, and I would
not have even noticed,
if it weren't for my
friend's story. I didn't
do anything about it, just
made mental note. My
eyes sometimes felt dry
and some mornings my
eyes were more puffy than
others, so then I considered
that all _three_ of these
things together might
be evidence of internal
inflammation.

The odd factor to me was that there were not any specific changes in my diet or routine because otherwise d could have a _mild_ _yeast_ _overgrowth_.

What's also different about me is the manner in which I approach problem solving. What I used to do is what a lot of people do: guess, tinker and perhaps make an appointment with an expert. Or what else?? _GOOGLE_ it!

These kinds of things are working from your __brain__. I've observed, especially with clients who come for colonics, and especially when it comes to correcting problems with health, __logic fails us.__

What I do is to ask myself If I actually _care_ about it. This strategy is based on the book, _Think and Grow Rich_, a classic about the power of visualization by Napoleon Hill. What he says, "if you care about it," it will expand:

For a lot of people, how *this* works is that CARE translates into worry.

what I care about → what I worry about

And then THAT expands.

HUMAN EMOTION is what expands, while LOGIC is more the mental structure which does not EXPAND, but just holds our interpretations in place.

This simple distinction, according to Napoleon Hill, makes all the difference in the world, which I apply to health AND in helping others to achieve better health.

If a person becomes ill, this is much harder to do.



worry suppresses improvement

This strategy is nothing
I stress very strongly
with my clients because
I've noticed a lot will
resist it or say that they've
already tried it, but
for me, it's my <u>first</u>
go to. It looked like this:



This usually takes me about
30 seconds to translate
a problem into a solution.

This tends to cause me to laugh at my problems:



What happens next, is that rather than ME getting out into left field, some kind of solution comes FROM left field while I DO nothing, especially not apply my own logic to the situation.

What happened with me is that "_intestinal parasites_" crept into my peripheral vision, I rejected it; it came closer, I considered it, then rejected it, then it SHOUTED, then I listened.

And I really can't care what anybody else thinks about it because it's just a story. This is also something which has required 15 years for me to unfold, so I respect that this isn't something you snap your fingers and everybody believes it.

This book will be going
from—

normal   to   "PARA" normal

Two car garage    land-scaping    dinner out    Public education

I will shortly get into it and will make every attempt to limit the time it takes to flip through this story to less than one hour, while the implications are many and complex. One can't just shout "WORMS!" in a crowded theater and let it go at that.

Here's roughly what you'll be getting into herewith because the time is _now_ to turn back and forget we ever had this conversation:

- Constipation is not today what it _was_ fifty years ago.

- The causes of constipation today are not what caused it fifty years ago.

- The notion that "the human body is self-cleansing" WAS true fifty years ago, is no longer true today.

- The notion of a high fiber diet plus drinking ample amounts of water to prevent or cure or treat a slow bowel is outdated.

- Both those and in the medical field AND in alternative health have not kept pace with the times. I don't care if your particular modality tradition is 5,000 years old, it's lost relevancy— particularly in the U.S. and increasingly elsewhere— with exceptions duly noted.

- The typical American is crawling with multiple types of parasites under their skin and large enough to view with the naked eye. This is from head to toe, including if you are one of those rare persons who has done multiple parasite cleanses — <u>head</u> <u>to</u> <u>toe</u>. It does not matter one iota whether you have traveled the world or if you are from <u>Muncie</u> and you've never left Indiana.

- How this has escaped notice for most all of human history, & have absolutely <u>no</u> clue. Honestly, I am embarrassed by the human race, Harvard Medical School, Mayo Clinic, Stanford, NASA, Perth, Tokyo, Berlin, and all the <u>rest</u> for <u>sleeping</u> on the job.
- It shouldn't require **me** to be put into this position to have

to write and draw
this out by hand,
no spell check, no
editor, no major publishing
house, no branding agency,
no publicity department,
no distribution agreements,
no book marketing genius,
no Dr. Oz invitations,
no press conferences,
no United Nations
backing, no World Health
Organization recognition,
no nothing. Just me.
Plus an amazing client possessed
by genius and a few more
willing to participate. Just _me_
with a cell phone camera.

Just me, submitting a
few itches and drynesses
to the grand scale of
the gods and the goddesses
going about their businesses
with nary a nod to
the gross complexities
happening beneath their
very feet, carelessly
tossing a rotten and slimy
fish in my direction from
far away in left field
as if granting me a nightmare
was the answer to my prayer!
So now you know.
It's too late to turn it
back.

# Introduction Part II

By way of quantifying and clarifying that none of this is my fault, National Geographic provides us some amazing photo and video documentation of parasitic life. And so does Discover magazine. These are readily available on YouTube so there's nothing covert or clandestine about it.

What's generally not known by the public is that parasitic species outnumber the regular kind we normally recognize as a bug or an animal by <u>4:1.</u> Most just don't float around in water so this does add a layer of complexity to <u>Noah</u> and <u>his ark</u>, which I may get into later. What these videos and articles reveal, because some of the videos I've watched multiple times, is that parasites are not just stealth, but totally creepy.

One type of parasitic wasp stalks a cockroach.



The wasp leaps out in surprise to sting the cockroach, which paralyzes it. With surgical precision, the wasp inserts its stinger-instrument into the victim's brain, then delicately probes and severs at the <u>exact</u> location where voluntary locomotion is controlled.

Then the wasp waits like a nurse for the anesthesia to totally take effect.



Not satisfied with mere appearances, the wasp severs an antennae to sample the roach's blood to be certain the anesthesia mix is JUST RIGHT.

This is straight out of the **Dexter** play book. Except this is a BUG with a built-in lab, surgical tool, a syringe, poison, and the perfect victim.

The wasp then leads this immobilized, docile victim to her den like a side of beef, where it lays her egg on the under-belly of the roach, which sleeps, but does not die, during gestation. The baby hatches as a larvae and knows exactly what to do—start eating. The larvae comes standard equipped with a sterilizing saliva, which it uses to preserve the now dead cockroach carcass, as the larvae matures daily until it leaves the nest to venture into the world.

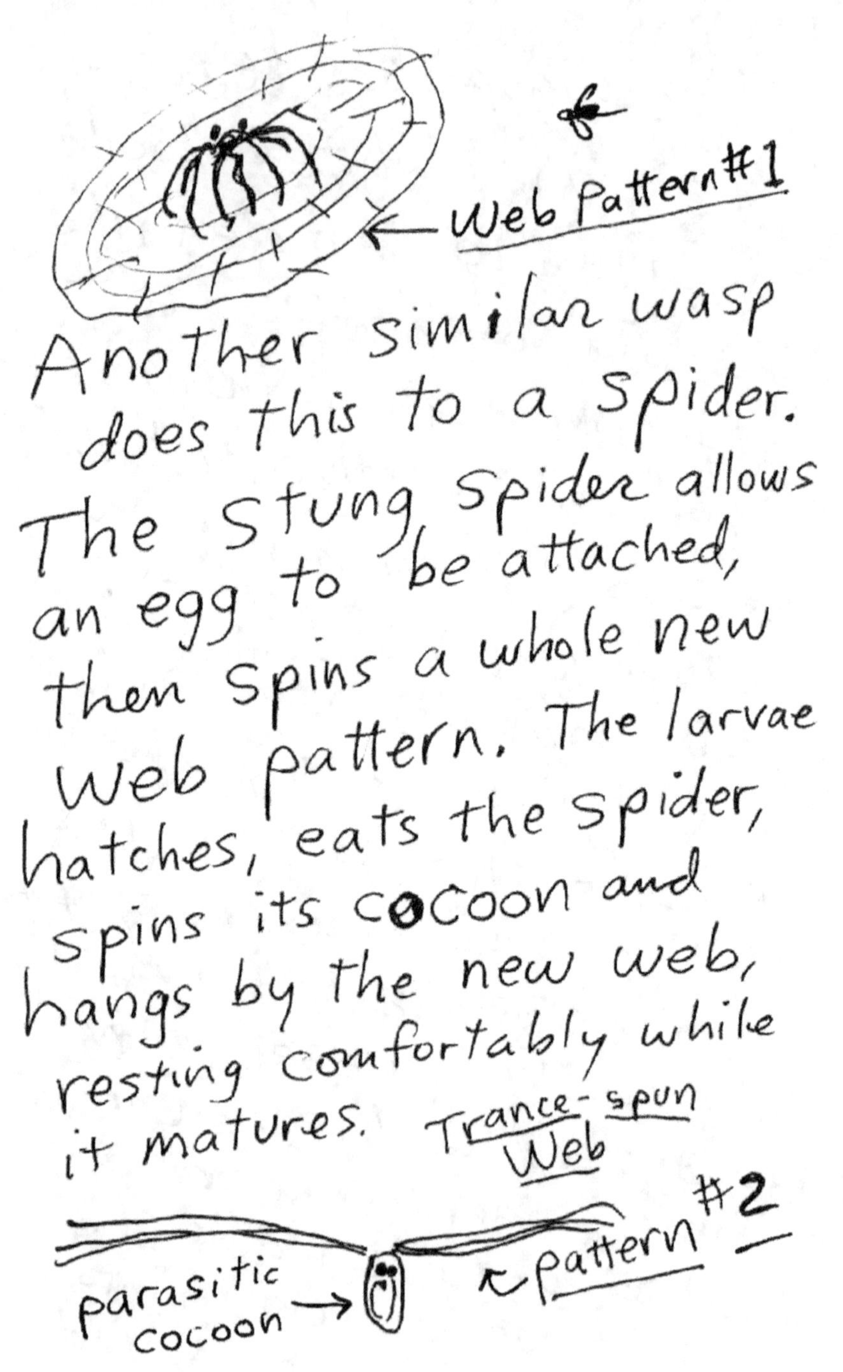


Another similar wasp does this to a spider. The stung spider allows an egg to be attached, then spins a whole new web pattern. The larvae hatches, eats the spider, spins its cocoon and hangs by the new web, resting comfortably while it matures.

Here's another brilliant
parasitic life cycle:

1) A mosquito dies,
drops to the ground.

infected
with
cyst
eggs →

2) A cricket comes
along and eats the
mosquito.

3) An egg hatches inside
the cricket, grows into
a hair-like worm, feeding
on the cricket, not killing it.

4) As if demon possessed,
the cricket throws itself
into water, which _the_
_worm_ requires to survive.

5.)



The cricket drowns as the worm unwinds-out saying, "Thanks for the ride!"

6.) Two worms spy each other, mate, lay eggs, which infect mosquito larvae growing in that same water. The eggs form protective cysts, the mosquito dies, and is eaten by a cricket.

There are many more examples, but you get the idea. In some cases, the larger parasites rely on smaller parasites in tandem. In other words, the _parasites_ possess parasites and in some cases, the parasites of the parasites have parasites. This can be a __Virus.__



Especially when scientists explore what's _behind_ parasitic mind control.

The larger parasite infects the body cavity.



while the virus disengages from the larger parasite and invades the brain.

Either way, parasites can affect brain chemistry, which can dramatically alter the host's behaviors.

Innovative scientists have described how an entire swamp ecosystem can be driven by parasitic control.

This kind of thing
could have implications
for Lyme disease
because ^human reactions can
be slight to extreme,
and treatment challenging,
and what if this could be
better understood if there's
an additional carrier parasite
not currently identified
as such?

Tick carries
borrelia
bacteria—
21 species can
cause Lyme.

If parasites have parasites, and they scientifically-proven do, then ticks might possibly be an intermediary stage between deer and humans, while the borrelia bacteria are actually passing between deer _liver_ _flukes_, which they commonly have, to human liver flukes.

Now I know almost nothing about Lyme disease, except that there is a lot of mystery surrounding it. Experts would point out that there is no way <u>liver flukes</u> could be connected to the life cycle of Lyme bacteria because Americans are <u>not</u> commonly infected with ~~Lyme~~ liver flukes, while they <u>are</u> with Lyme bacteria.

That makes perfect sense
if you are basing _the_ _number_
of liver flukes in Americans
based on _diagnosis._ As
I mentioned earlier, we
have thrown our _thinking_ _caps_
out the window. We are
as stupid as the village
idiot.   The job we've been
given is to remove poop
from people all day long.

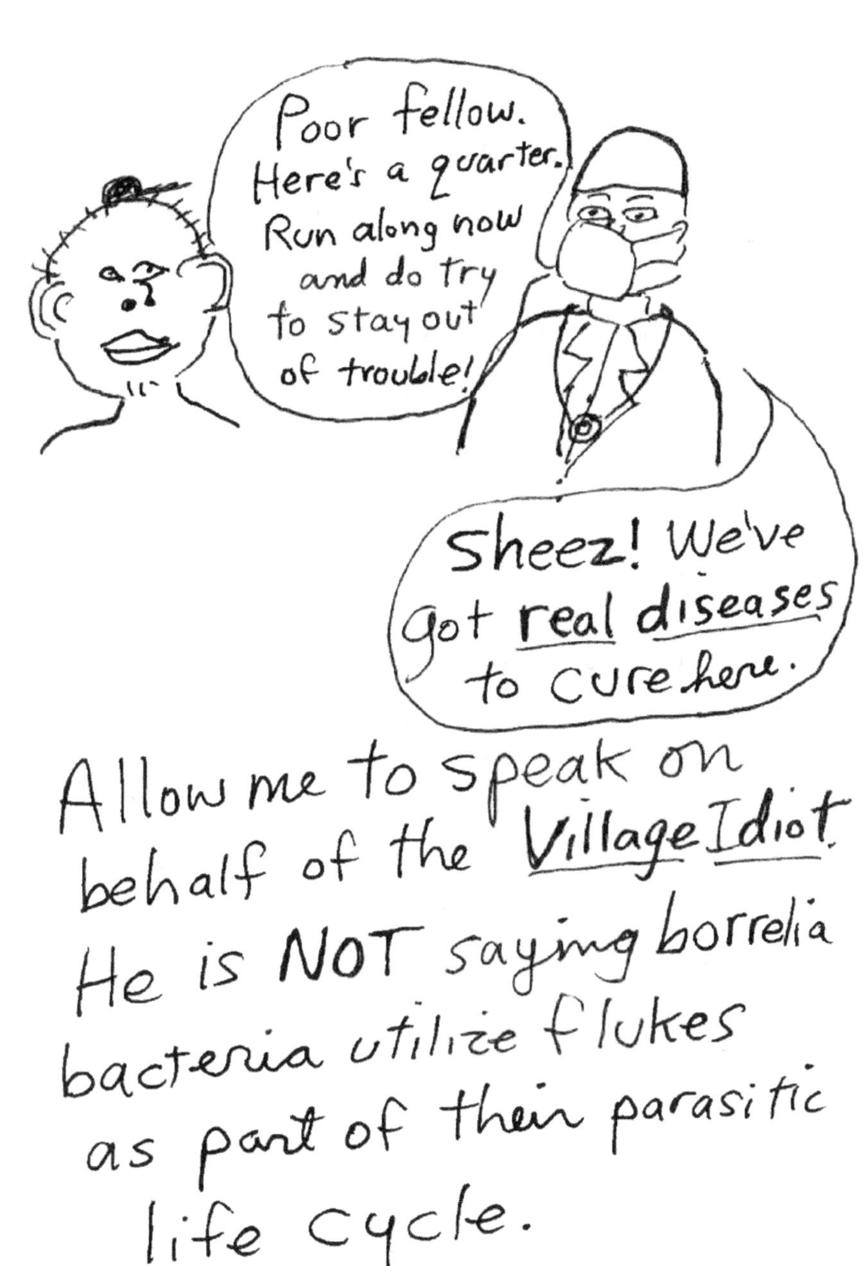


Allow me to speak on behalf of the Village Idiot. He is NOT saying borrelia bacteria utilize flukes as part of their parasitic life cycle.

Village Idiot Boy _is_ merely saying, that when somebody, _anybody_, is on some kind of a parasite cleanse, _he_ sees <u>WORMS</u>.

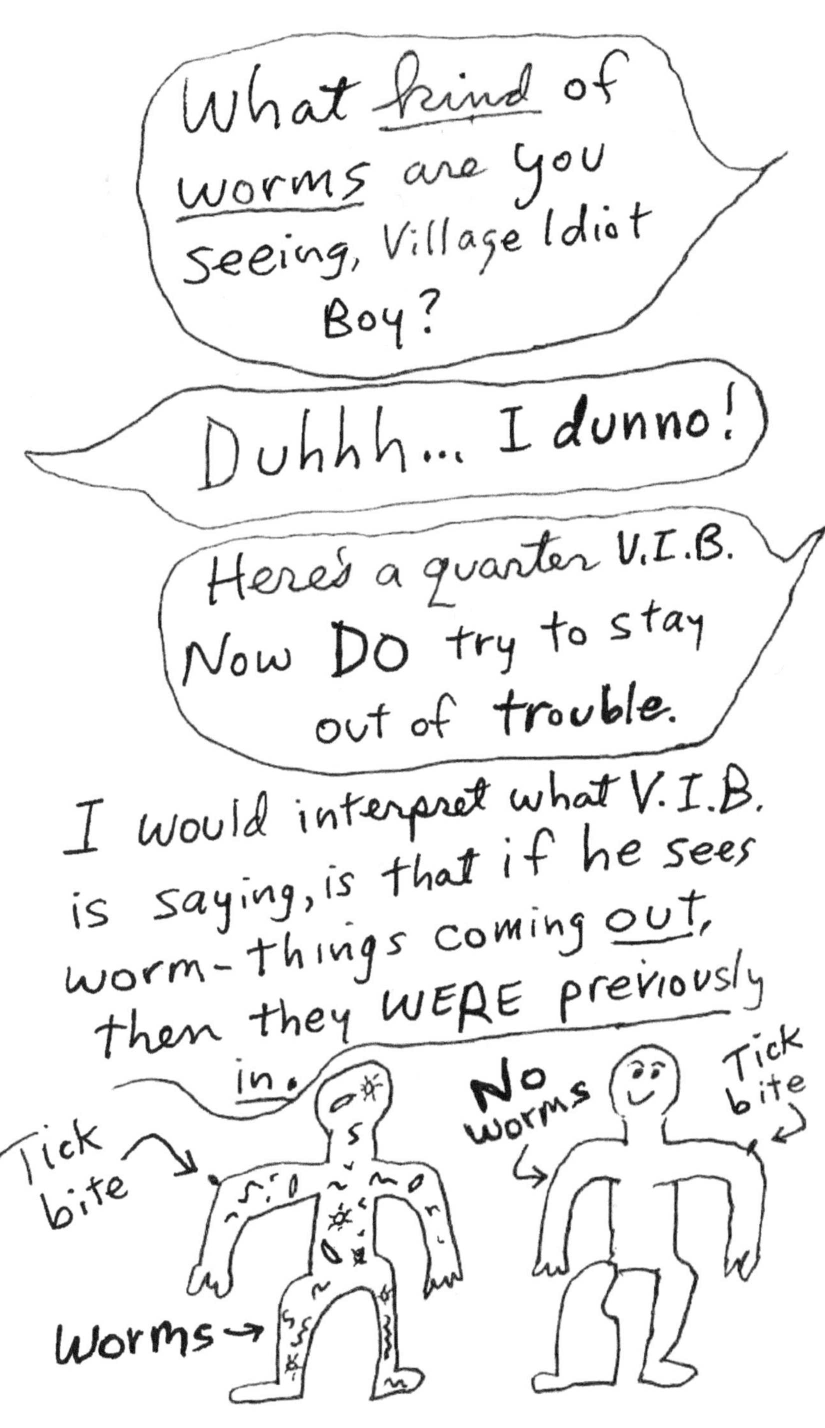

What kind of worms are you seeing, Village Idiot Boy?

Duhhh... I dunno!

Here's a quarter V.I.B. Now DO try to stay out of trouble.

I would interpret what V.I.B. is saying, is that if he sees worm-things coming out, then they WERE previously in.

Tick bite

Tick bite

No worms

Tick bite

Worms →

And that a human
infested with multiple
species of worm-like
things MIGHT react
differently from a human
infested with **no** worms.
So if we (just briefly)
shifted the medical
paradigm to the diagram
that 100.00% of Americans
do have worms, maybe
that could explain
part of the mystery
surrounding the understanding
and treatment of
Lyme disease.

We'd like to see the expert medical folks really <u>stretch</u> and just consider it, and not j<u>ust</u> related to Lyme disease, and they jussst can't do it. They are physically and emotionally unable to take one, two, three steps to just glance at what Village Idiot Boy sees, because it's just not possible that worms living inside Americans could be for real.

This is when the
realization strikes!
The medical paradigm
is an assembly line
which produces <u>products.</u>
Everything around us
is saying <u>YOU WANT IT</u>!

But we could say the exact same about alternative health care:

No matter what anybody calls it, your health can be defined as a _consumer_ pie chart.

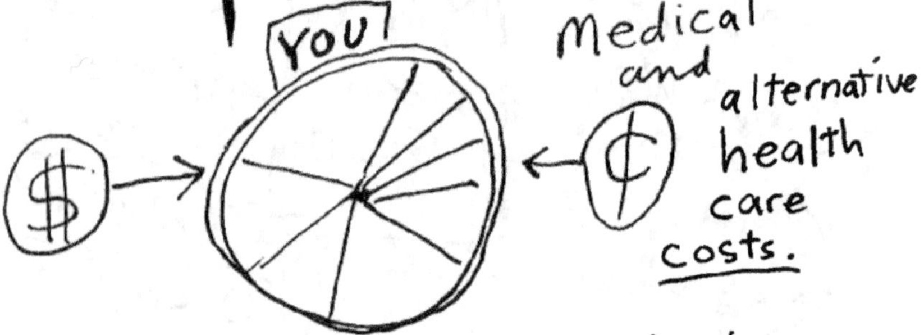

Another way to look at it is _mind shares:_

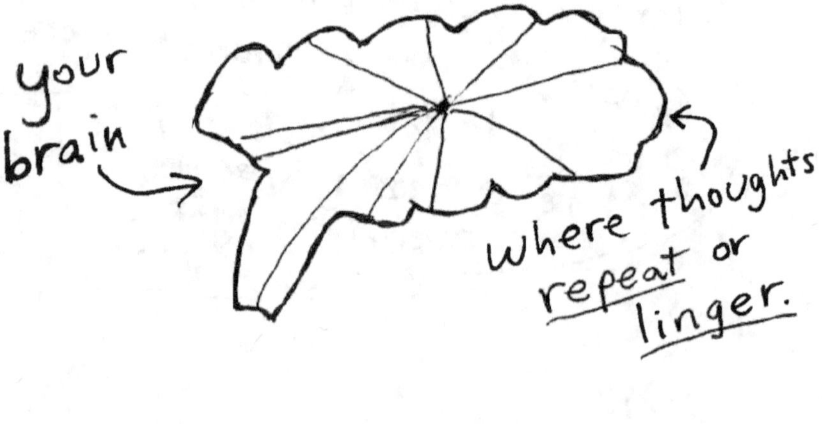

This is not much different than a parasitic wasp going into your brain and severing your voluntary locomotion control.

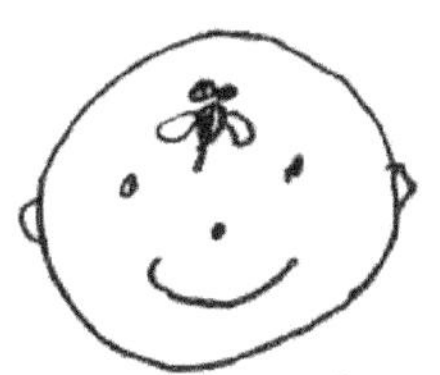

Then clipping your antennae and sampling to check how it's all working.

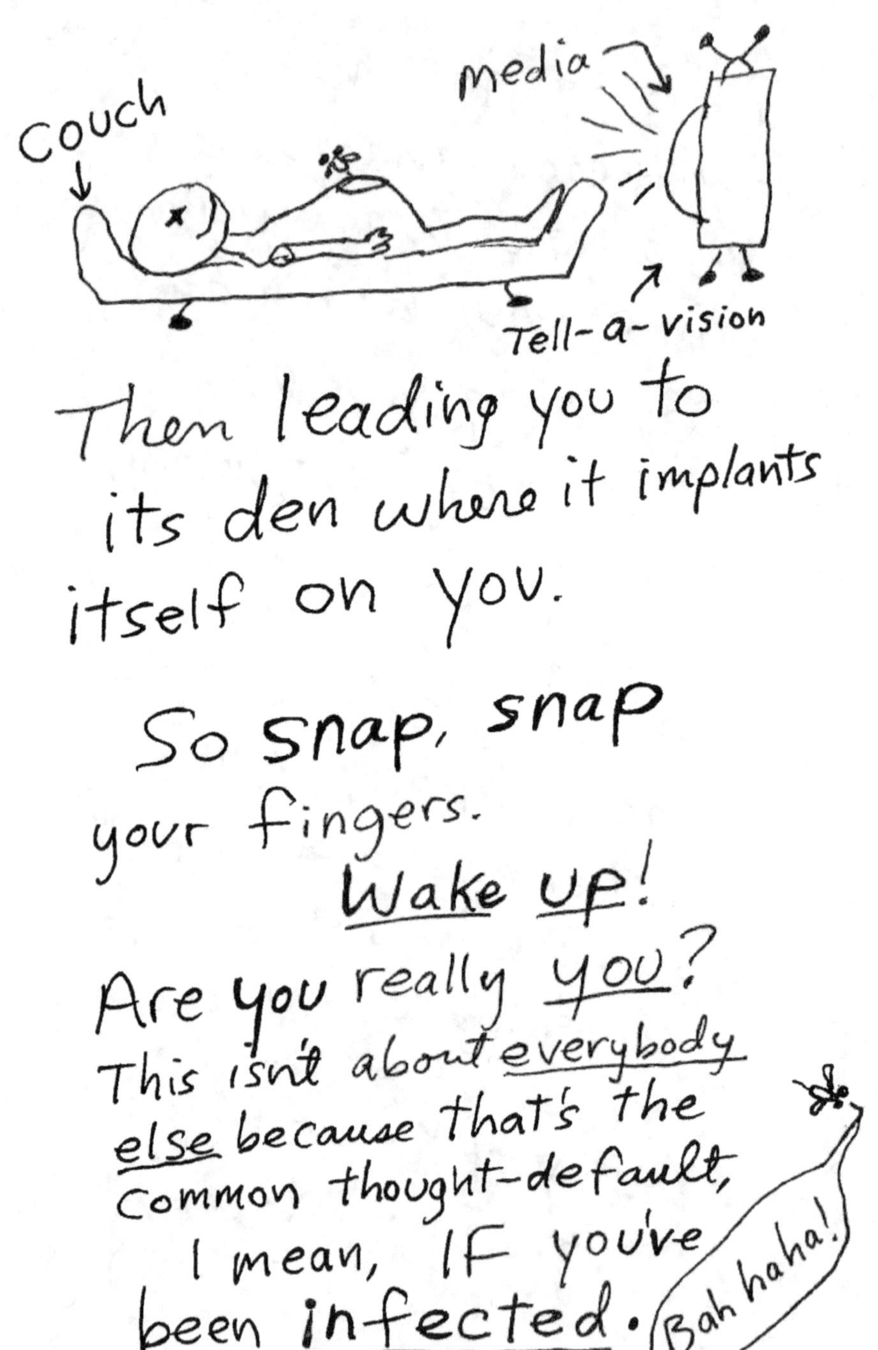


Then leading you to its den where it implants itself on you.

So snap, snap your fingers. <u>Wake up</u>!

Are you really <u>you</u>? This isn't about <u>everybody else</u> because that's the common thought-default, I mean, IF you've been <u>infected</u>.

<u>Introduction Part III</u>

The topic of human parasites can be addressed on many levels.

It can be a lot like <u>ghosts</u>.



You would believe in ghosts if you yourself had seen one. But then, if somebody else told you THEY saw a ghost, you could feel <u>skeptical</u>.

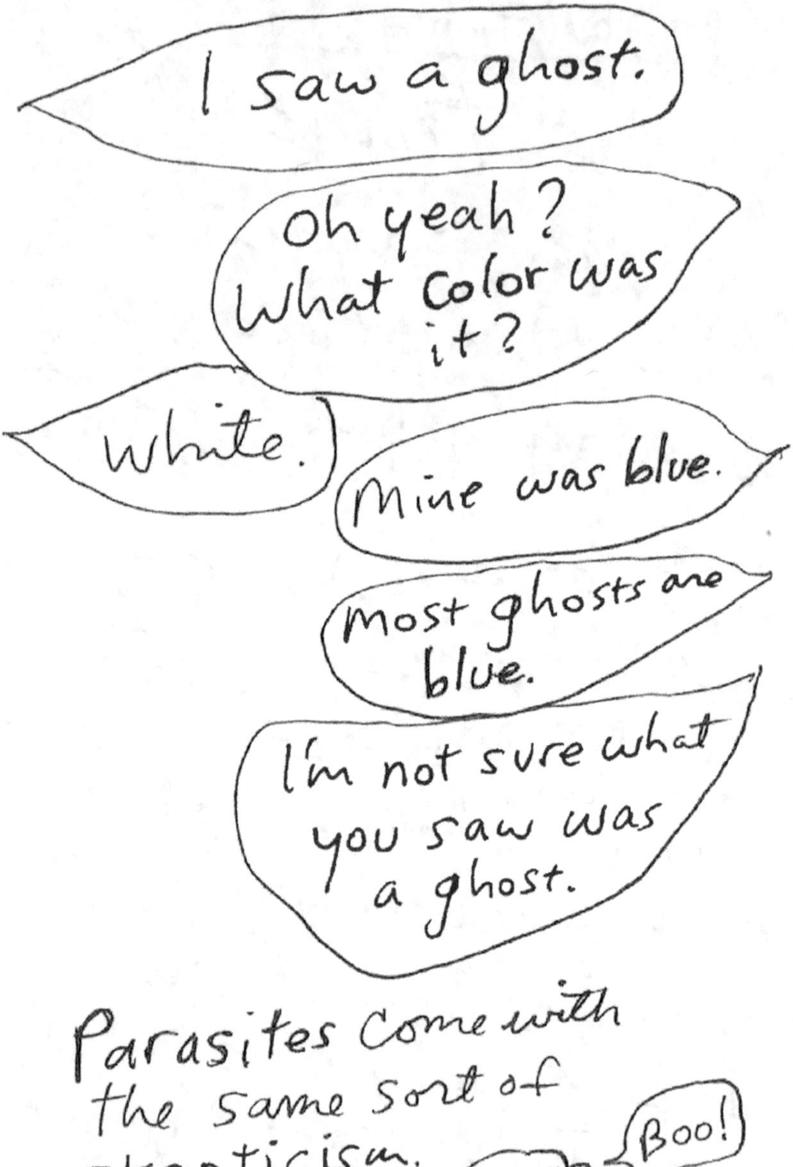

Parasites come with the same sort of skepticism.

Our culture doesn't offer the context to discuss parasites.



Certainly not at dinner.



It won't come up on the tennis court or on the golf course.

Even at the doctor's office it could come across as a bit wacky.

Despite that the
opiate addiction crisis
is all over the news,
if it hasn't touched you
directly, it's almost
difficult to believe.
It makes sense mostly within the ~~as a~~
larger national pattern of
illness, and pain, and CHRONIC.

If we are coming to grips, let's not pretend that the current, widespread state of health in America is anything to <u>celebrate</u>.

And let's not GLOSS OVER that the news most Americans read about health ~~are~~ is deeply rooted in the <u>PRESS RELEASE</u>.

Corporate H.Q. → PR Dept. → Proper Channels → Media → Newsroom → mass dissemination → Google it → Down the rabbit hole

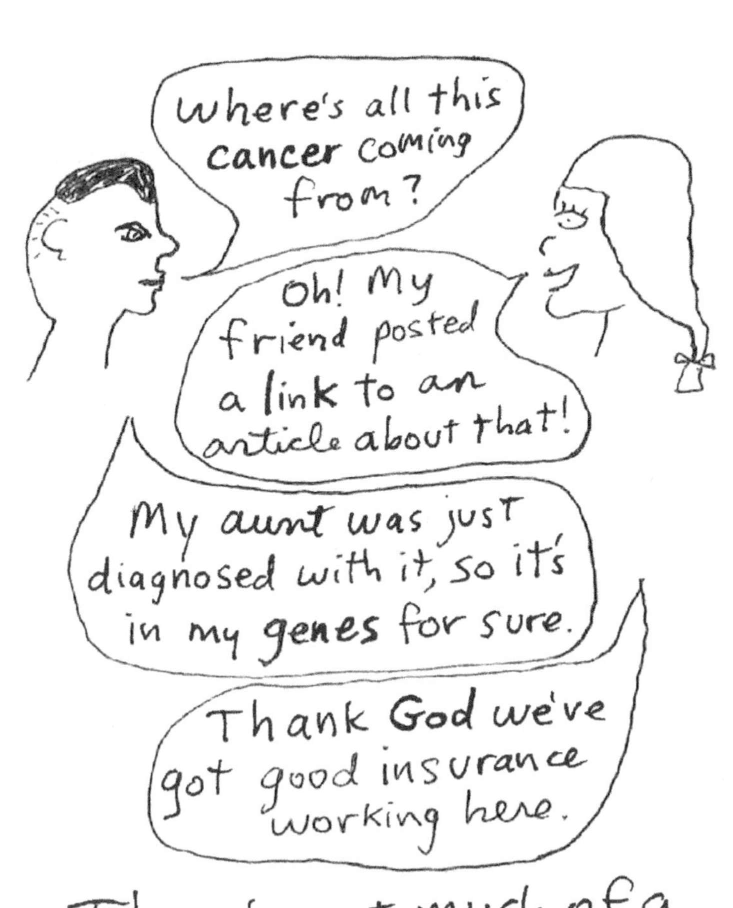


There's not much of a reason to delve deeper than that. Plus—our attention spans are shortening. Or at least, you know, I read that somewhere.

Now if everything was just **normal**, it wouldn't matter. This is because we tend to operate our critical thinking around <u>normalacy</u>.

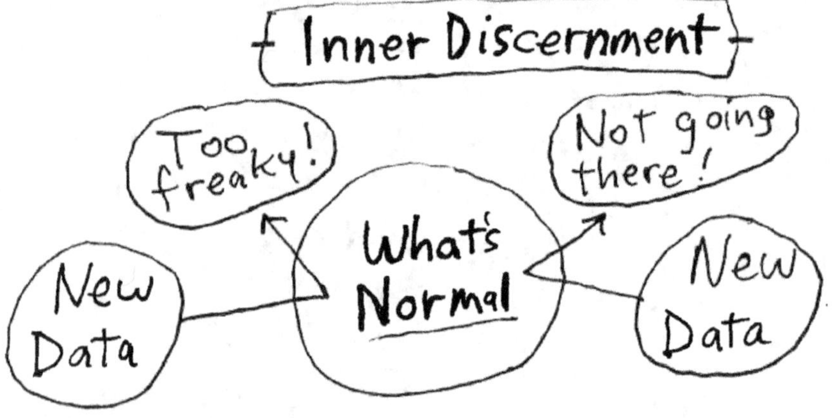


This possibly could inversely flip if the new normal is the "not-normal."

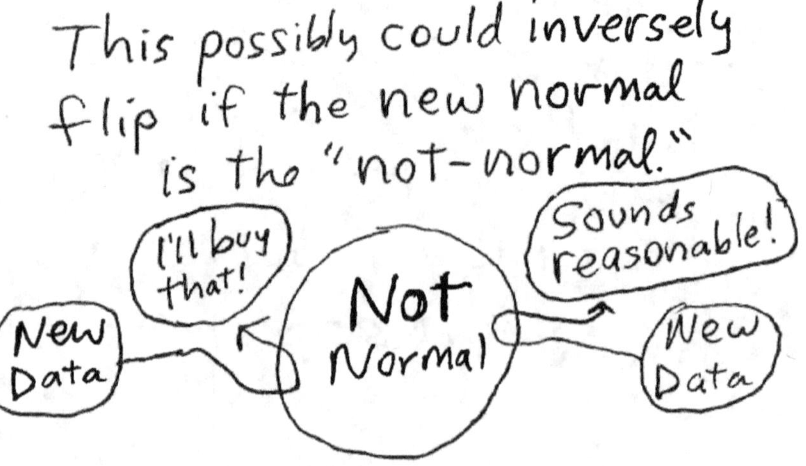

You would THINK our beliefs center around cognition, or what's mental, but it's actually more like a hockey game.



Each side wants to pack the stands with fans who can together create a fever pitch resonation which can <u>force</u> the puck into the goal. (Those on the fence don't belong there.)

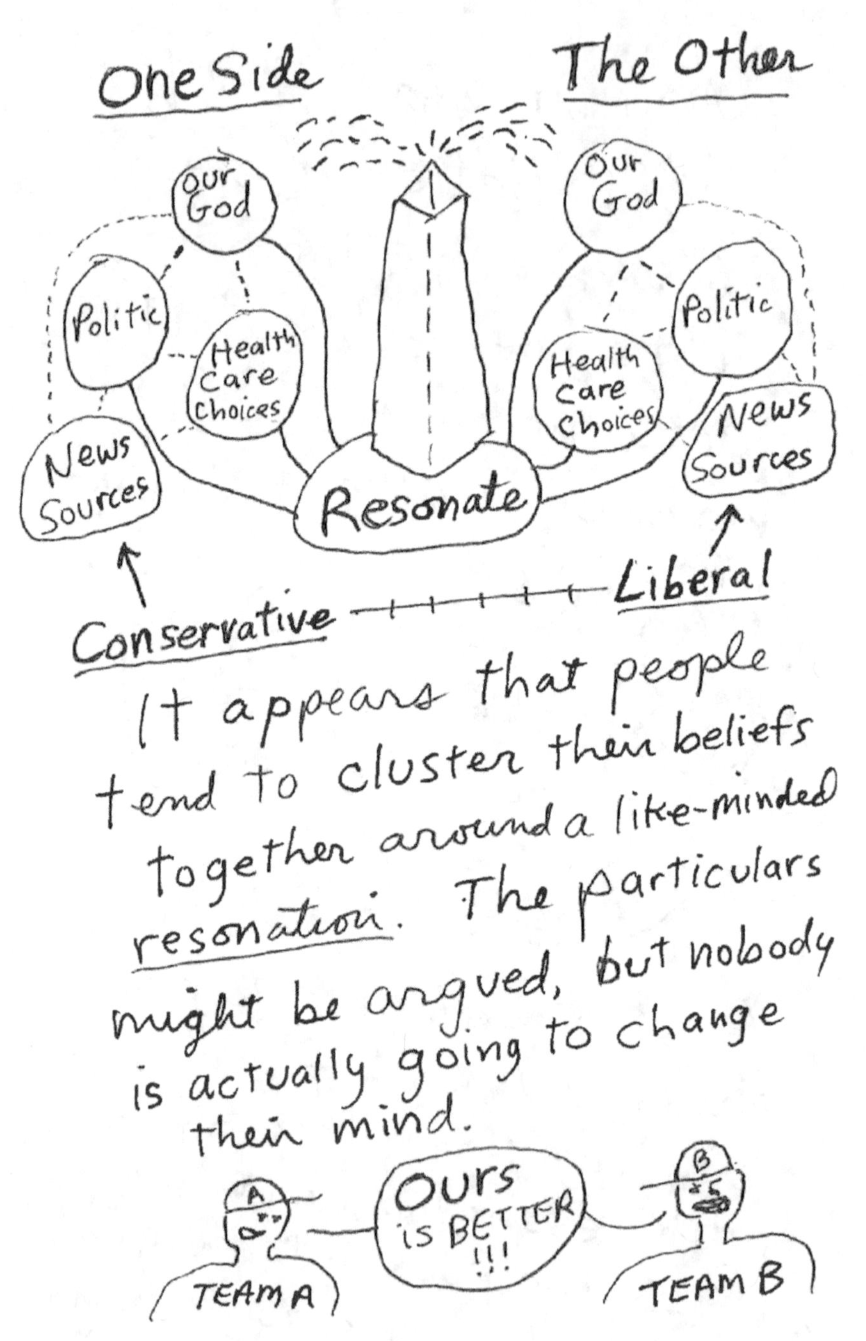


It appears that people tend to cluster their beliefs together around a like-minded resonation. The particulars might be argued, but nobody is actually going to change their mind.

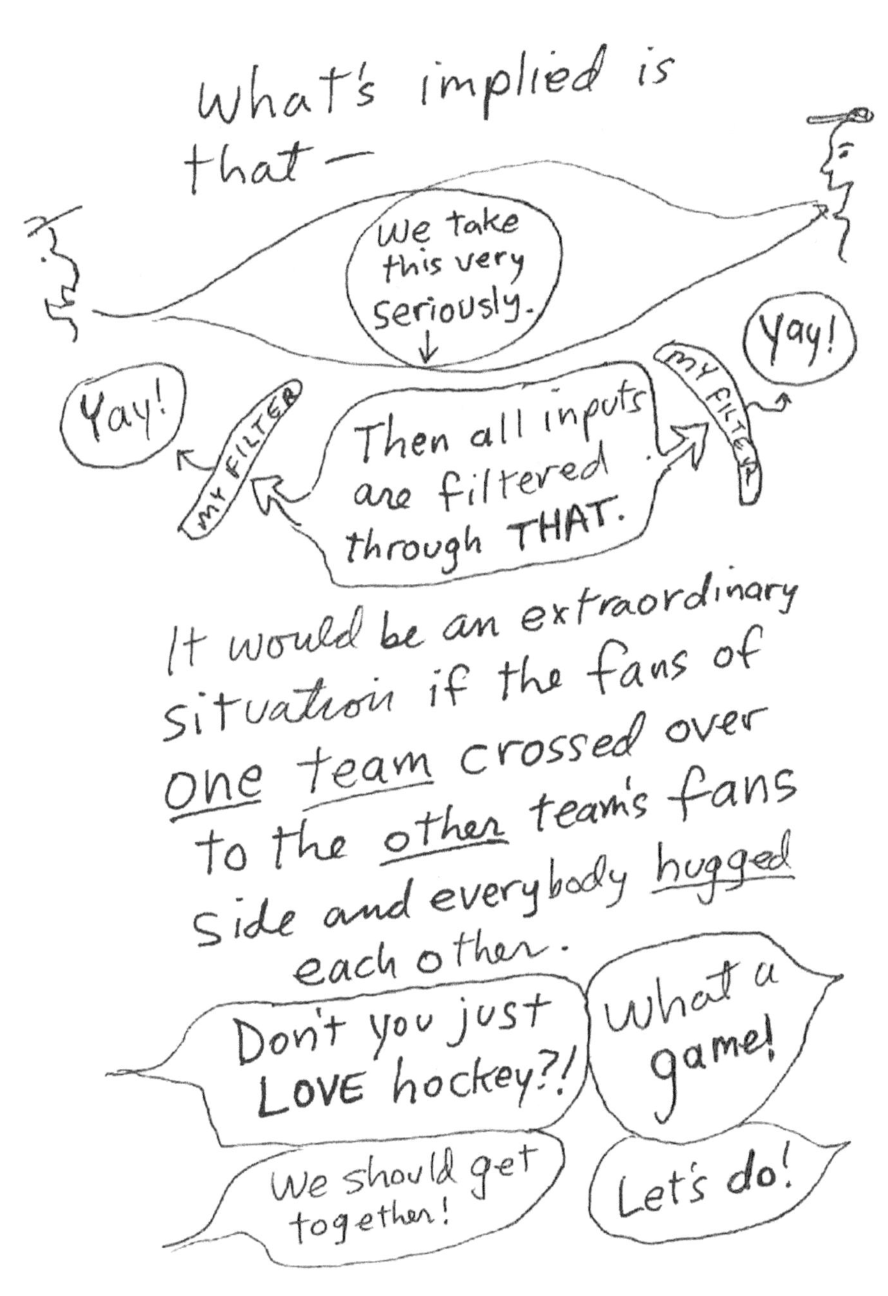

What's implied is that—
We take this very seriously.
Yay!
MY FILTER
Then all inputs are filtered through THAT.
MY FILTER
Yay!
It would be an extraordinary situation if the fans of one team crossed over to the other team's fans side and everybody hugged each other.
Don't you just LOVE hockey?!
What a game!
We should get together!
Let's do!

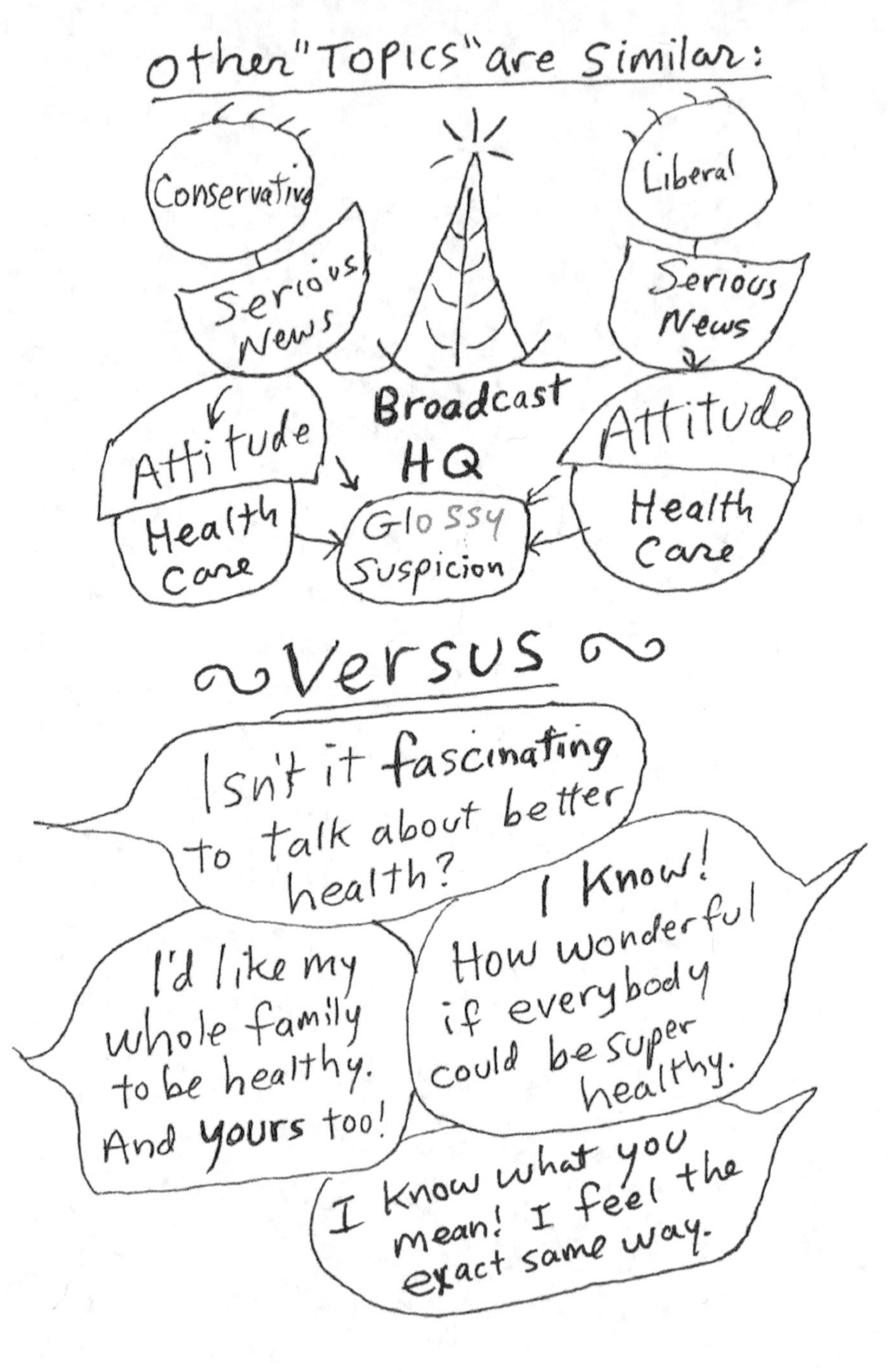

other "TOPICS" are similar:
Conservative
Liberal
Serious News
Serious News
Attitude
Broadcast HQ
Attitude
Health Care
Glossy Suspicion
Health Care
~ Versus ~
Isn't it fascinating to talk about better health?
I'd like my whole family to be healthy. And yours too!
I know! How wonderful if everybody could be super healthy.
I know what you mean! I feel the exact same way.

But then there's:



So it's tricky because if a person is going to write about **parasites;** no matter what, it's on the outer fringes of what's fun. This is why contrast and absurdity are the best tools to communicate:

Scott W. Webb

Author Bio

I'm listening to an audio recording of the autobiography of Donna Karan, about half way into it. If you don't know who she is, she's a bit of a celebrity fashion designer and I had no idea how thrilling fashion could be. I'm at the point in her story where she's come through about 20 years of constant multitasking, like talking on the phone while receiving a pedicure, eating lunch, and sorting through fabric swatches she had brought back from a trip to Bali. Her frenetic pace is beginning to transition more inward. She describes observing her own intuition and sensitivity as a particular rock on the beach "speaks" to her or the trees she is drawn to, which she hugs. She carries a potato in a bag to show others the quality of tone she hopes to duplicate. I identify with her insatiable curiosity.

Meanwhile she is
beginning to spin counter
to the increasing corporate
mindset encroaching upon
her **creative space**.
     The focus of this
book is on human parasites,
while what's just as relevant
is the BIG PICTURE of
you. I've shown clients photos
of wormy things coming
out in their colonic water
and noticed that the
conversation speeds up.
A kind of panic sets in.
If they too have worms

living inside of _them_, they want them OUT. NOW! Like _Yesterday!_

But it doesn't work like that. You can run fast with the rest of your life, but with removing internal parasites, it requires to slooow down.

As Donna Karan's financial security was more and more guaranteed, she then observed the truism that _money_ can't buy health.

That comes as an epiphany when you possess money and somebody close to you becomes ill. So we want to know — is there some other tangible that DOES buy health? Seriously, _what_ could that be? (It might be better to buy it when you don't need it, like when it's marked down on sale.)

Articles and books were published decades ago about the health damages from candida overgrowth, and it's taken till recently to bubble up into the mainstream.

Human parasites in the form of **WORMS** is on the cutting edge of quackery. Until recently, I too believed that. As I started to see what is going on, it was shocking to me — even tears flew from my eyes in front of my client, while after calming down a little, perhaps

it is good to slow down
and for me to go into
more detail.
My story is nothing
like Donna Karan's story.
For one, I have absolutely
no fashion sense. She is
New York City and I'm like
cornfield Midwest. My
mother's family came from
Nebraska off the farm
and my father's family
history runs through a
tiny town outside Kansas
City. My parents have

the unusual distinction
of dating (off & on) since
the 8th grade. This was
in Chicago, post Depression,
World War II era, a time
when good health was a
given. "Candida overgrowth"
wasn't even a concept.
If a family had a pet,
nobody considered that
it had worms and
Grandma might have been
testy, but never, ever
thought to have parasites!
Even when I grew up, I
never knew of a KID
who had <u>cancer</u>.

After college, my father
enlisted in the Air Force
and was trained to be
a pilot. About this time
my mom and dad were
married and they lived
in Morocco where my dad
was stationed. After his
service, they returned to
Chicago and he entered
into the field of commercial
refrigeration, grocery store
design and equipment sales.
In 1965, he became partners
in a commercial refrigeration
company located in Rockford,
Illinois, where I grew
up.

My older brother has an M.D. degree in optometry and today is in private practice in Janesville, Wisconsin. My younger brother got his MBA at Northwestern University's Kellogg School and most of his career has been in the health insurance industry. My younger sister graduated from the University of Wisconsin, has five children, and lives in Lake Placid, Florida.

The reason I mention these things is because

there is **nothing** in my background that suggests that one day I would grow up to become a <u>colon hygienist</u>. And then put together a book about human <u>parasites.</u>

One of my interests as a young adult was in Christianity. I could stay up all night talking about it and sometimes did. When I was 16, I went on a summer youth missions trip to Alaska where we built two cabins at a Bible

Camp and the following summer helped to build a small cinder block church on the Caribbean island of Dominica. I was driven by the idea that life is short and therefore it would be better to attend to _eternal_ things. My college education also revolved around this same theme, graduating from Wheaton College outside Chicago with a B.A. degree in philosophy.

For my language requirement to graduate, I studied Ancient Greek in a summer intensive and made straight A's.

Learning Greek – or at least figuring out what it took to make straight A's in Greek class, was my best preparation for becoming a colon hygienist. Yes, believe it or not, poop isn't just "poop" because there are many <u>fine</u> <u>distinctions</u>. You begin knowing nothing about it, then must make <u>sense</u> of the <u>minuscia</u>.

After college, I visited
my older brother and his
wife who were both
stationed on Kodiak Island,
Alaska, in the Coast Guard.
I ended up staying for
8 months because, by
chance, I was hired
to be the advertising
manager at the town's
newspaper. After saving
$3,000, which was a small
fortune to me, I quit,
flew to visit a friend
in Oregon, bought an

old Volvo 122S, then took
a two month road trip
up and down California.
I spent the winter months
in Seattle working at a
restaurant. In the spring
I wanted to get back to
Alaska. I had saved just
enough money to buy a used
1973 Honda CL360 motorcycle
and a ferry ticket to get
me to Haines, AK. It
was early April when we
left WA. North beyond Juneau,
it started to <u>SNOW.</u>
        By Haines, it was
an all out blizzard!

My boots weren't waterproof.
I had made sandwiches
for my trip which had
been stuffed into two
bread bags and I used
those bags on my _feet_ to
cover my boots and I
stuffed a _Seattle Times_
newspaper up my coat
as a wind breaker.
The blizzard lasted
three days so I was
stuck in Haines and
couldn't afford a motel
room. I explained my
situation to a guy at

a sandwich shop and
he was kind enough
to let me sleep in his
storage shed for no
charge and then I
drove to Anchorage,
which took me 3 days
across a moonscape of
snow, with additional
kindnesses extended to
me all along the way.
I spent the rest of
the decade of the 1980s
living in Anchorage
and worked seven years

in advertising at The Anchorage Daily News, got married in 1984 and we had a son born in 1986 and a daughter in 1988.

Again, the reason I explain this is so you know that I'm not some kind of a parasite-obsessed nut. Plus, I like ~~seek out~~ frontiers.

The young woman I married was a singer and songwriter which is why we ended up moving to Nashville in 1990. Since then, I've met lots of people who have been to Alaska and most went there on a cruise ship. When it comes to taking some sort of action to cleanse parasites from the human body, there's not really a cruise ship type of methodology to take you there. It's more like you show up in a port town during a blizzard driving a blizzard driving a motorcycle and you realize your feet will soon be soaked and frozen, so you look around for something that might help to waterproof your shoes. It's going to be a difficult journey, but you might find yourself singing along the way to nobody at the top of your lungs. This is going to be what you could call an ADVENTURE. I mean, learning more about PARASITES!

I'd like to point out
that if you _do_ have
worm-like parasites
living inside your organs
and tissues, your
back is against the wall,
same as mine has been.
The way forward is
forward, and no
matter what, it will be
the _road_ _less_ _traveled_.
when I learned
that some people were
swallowing turpentine
to kill their parasites,

I had to stop and really think about what people are doing. Turpentine is the Wild West of holistic therapies. If it's a kind of snake oil, it's the snakiest! Research it yourself,* of course, but if you do try it, be sure to make a toast. "To your health!"

After you get used to the idea that weird wormy things could infest you right here in America, you will likely reverse course and think it's all a <u>hoax.</u>

<u>* I accept no liability.</u>

The problem is, there's a bit of a HOAX in everything. If Donna Karan invested her **all** into fashion, I've spent a good part of my life exploring and penetrating through what's commonly considered hoax. To me, it's like Greek to say that money can't buy health if you don't know **what** will. Like many things, it's a **riddle**.

If you want to **buy health,** solve the riddle!

We will know you
are solving the
riddle when we see
the bread bags over
your shoes.

---

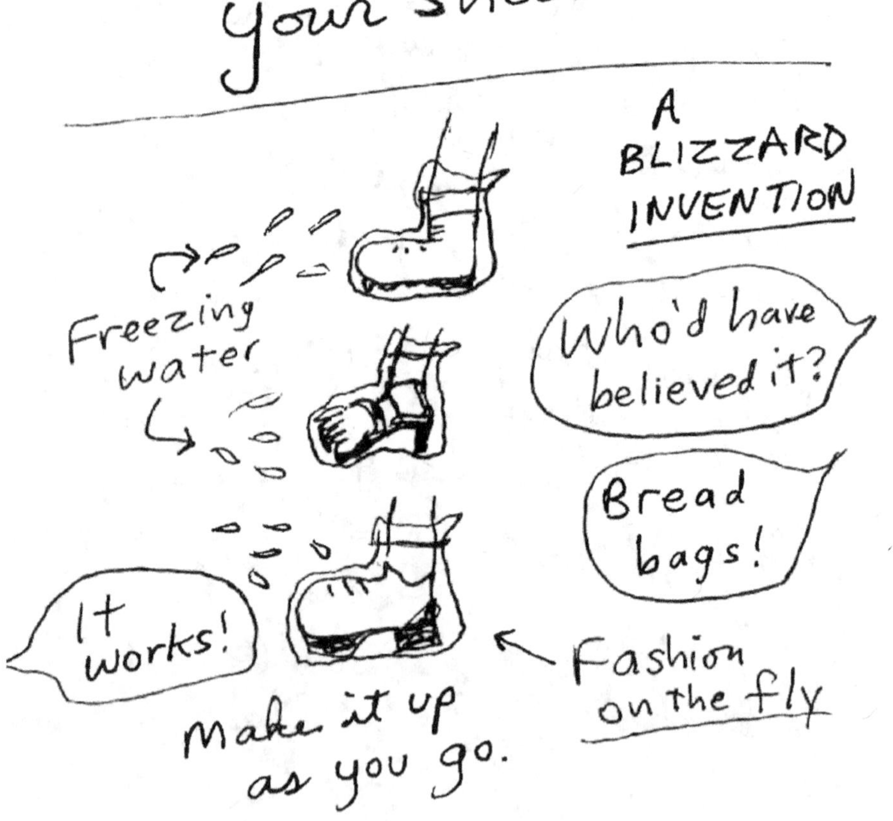

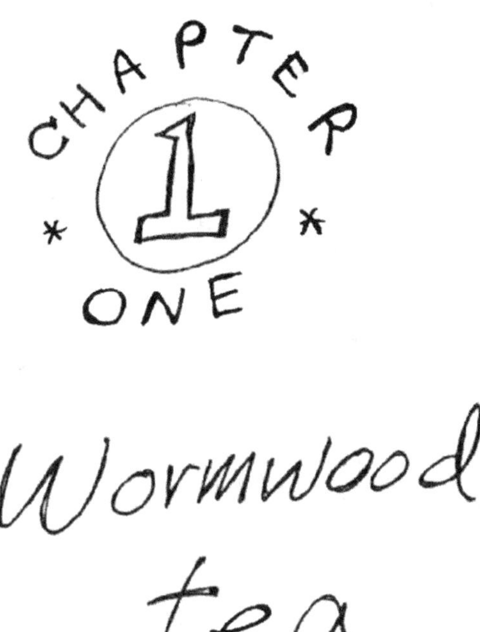


# Wormwood tea

One highly trusted source of health information and break through stuff is the Dr. Oz Show. I myself don't own a television, but as a colon hygienist, I do a lot of laundry. The laundromat has a television and sometimes I'll catch The Dr. Oz Show for a few minutes. My impression is that Dr. Oz is super likeable and I like him too.
However, the show's information is often lacking

$\longrightarrow$

as he presents himself.
as a kind of alternative
holistic M.D. blend, backed
by clinical research and
guest expertise.

One show covered
parasites and as of this
moment, it's on YouTube.
It's called, "Parasites In
America." Feel free to
watch it and follow along.

#1 The beginning
is like a horror movie
trailer or a PARODY
of a horror movie
trailer.

#2 Now we see the studio audience reacting.



#3 Now we are introduced to an M.D. gastroenterologist who is completely calm, educated, and well spoken. What we want to notice is the contrast between the doctor and the studio audience.

#4   The gastroenterologist expert guest states that actually, parasites are a <u>more common</u> problem <u>than we know</u>. She cites one study of <u>chronic fatigue</u> patients, that 46% of them were discovered to "have parasites behind their symptoms." The question to be asked is, "Do most gastroenterologists treating chronic fatigue believe <u>parasites</u> can be the <u>cause</u> of CFS?" If so, patients would be <u>treated</u> for such.

This doctor walks us through three parasite remedies: eating garlic, drinking wormwood tea, and consuming half a cup of papaya seeds daily for up to two weeks.

Again, **is <u>this</u>** what doctors treating **CFS** are actually recommending to their patients? Maybe not. A lot of people would say—

Something else we want
to consider is—
How many TV viewers
are actually SUFFERING
with chronic fatigue?
Wouldn't they be on
the edge of their seats,
full of trust and hope
that Dr. Oz would not
steer them wrong?
The audience watches
the two doctors sip
wormwood tea and
their reactions tell us
this is the first time
they've tried it.
YUK!

We are not really certain whether wormwood tea is a treatment for <u>CFS</u> or just for the prevention of "parasites." Dr. Oz tells everybody that this is <u>easy</u>, but what he's really saying is that he <u>himself</u> doesn't drink it.

The gastroenterologist says wormwood tea kills round worms. It paralyzes them and they lay less eggs, which reduces the spread of worms to others.

Wait a minute!

I am assuming that most Americans do their #2 business into a TOILET. Then wouldn't it travel via the sewer system to a <u>sanitization</u> facility? What does she mean, "<u>Less</u> EGGS?" If a round worm was inside of us, wouldn't we want <u>NO</u> EGGS? How many eggs hatching would we need to be completely reinfested? Plus, the discussion about <u>chronic</u> <u>fatigue</u> stopped, so do <u>round</u> <u>worms</u> <u>cause</u> CFS?

Then the guest doctor goes on to explain that if you don't like the tea, you can buy wormwood as a _tincture_, and then she says— "which can be added to…" BUT she stops talking because she realizes that she actually _doesn't know_ _what_ you'd add wormwood tincture **to**. But she's fast on her feet and _distracts_ _us_ by saying she'd like to "try some wormwood tea too!"
NICE!

When I Google "chronic"
+ "fatigue" + "parasite,"
what I pull up is <u>WebMD.</u>
(Now <u>there's</u> a reputable
source of straight talk.)
Click on that and we
learn :<sup>Quote</sup> " Doctors <u>don't</u>
<u>know</u> what causes chronic
fatigue syndrome. In some
cases, CFS symptoms
start after a <u>viral</u> illness."

So if I am <u>seriously</u>
looking for answers about
CFS and I've watched the
Dr. Oz Show, then read
about it on WebMD, I'm
confused, down the <u>rabbit hole.</u>

I mentioned earlier that my grandparents were born and raised in rural Nebraska. The story goes that one evening, decades ago, my grandmother got creative in the kitchen and made a pizza for supper. My grandfather picked up a slice and threw it against the wall. He said: "I want a little meat, some potatoes, some vegetables, and that's IT."

When I grew up, that's mostly how we ate, too.

If something alternative was being served, it came with some fanfare, like "We are making MEXICAN tonight," or "We're having lasagna!" If we went out for Chinese, it was like, wow, Chinese! But the basic structure of diet was ingrained — a little meat, a little potato and some vegetables. Fast food fit nicely into this same model, the vegetables being a little onion, pickles, ketchup and mustard. Once I became an adult myself and was exposed to various "more healthy" dietary options, my thought was — somebody is trying to make a buck. A drink made from wheat grass? Look at the price. That's pure profit!

I viewed illness in the same skeptical light, partially because in my family, and around our neighborhood, people didn't get sick for more than a day or two. I equated something like "chronic fatigue syndrome" as an excuse for _LAZINESS_. If you're feeling tired, you go to bed earlier the next night or you _slap_ something on your face, shut up, and keep going.

So something like _COLONICS_ was _way_

outside my general idea
of what a sane person
would **PAY** for.

So there's something
else at play and it's often
based on considerations one
must ease into. When
I was invited to study
colon hydrotherapy, it was
something I did on a lark.
I did not expect to return
for a second training class
and when I did open a
professional colon cleaning
office with the woman I
trained with, it was more
her idea, not mine.

Then when I would have
a new client come in
and start telling me about
all their illnesses, my
thought was — you really
ought to see a DOCTOR.
For me, there was a huge
Category divide between
what colon hygiene could
do and what a doctor
would do.  This was
inbred : If you are sick,
                 truly
go to a doctor.
        what happened was
that people would come
in, sit down, tell me

102

about some kind of
illness symptoms they had,
and <u>had</u> gone to a
doctor, and were told either
there was nothing found
to be wrong or whatever
the doctor had prescribed
hadn't helped AND they'd
gone to a <u>second</u> and <u>third</u>
doctor, plus a specialist,
and they'd often almost
BEG me — " Do you think
a <u>colonic</u> will help me?"
<u>My response</u>:
" I seriously doubt it."
They'd always do a
colonic anyway so it

was a series of experiments that I wasn't organizing. Sometimes the resulting benefits were profound and somewhat confounding because it was like, **How can this be?** Especially with rashes and skin conditions. At first I'd tell my clients, "There's no way in hell a colonic will help for that," but then it would. And after a year of that, or two or three years, just when I was mostly optimistic that a colonic COULD help with this or that, it wouldn't help. What I'd say to clients was, "If you think it will help, let's give it a try."

Now up until this point in my life (in my early forties), I'd never read a single book about health. That changed. I was reading about health constantly because I wanted to know what was going on.

I mean, what seemed to be happening

was a massive DISCONNECT between the health issues facing LOTS of Americans and the way doctors were approaching it. I'd have clients explaining their symptoms and ailments and CRYING. At first, I was responding, "Don't come in here for a <u>colonic</u> and start crying." But then in time I could see, these weren't stupid people, something <u>WAS</u> haywire. Sometimes

it was the opposite.
A client might say:
"I'm a cancer survivor and
all my doctors and
nurses were wonderful."
The thing is, I don't
really care either way.
I just want people to
solve their problems as
effectively as possible
and if there's anything I
can do to help, I will.
So if I'm walking
through the laundromat
and notice that the Dr. Oz
show is on, I'll stop
for a minute and
watch.

My main thing is to say **HUH!** Sometimes I might say, "That's interesting," or "that's a crock," which I <u>can</u> say because nobody is asking my opinion. But when you've actually studied on the topic of health and experimented, whether intentionally or not, you start coming across illness in the news <u>a lot</u> and you start saying a lot to yourself — "That's a crock," and you want to be careful with it or you can just walk around feeling mad and critical.

The best way for me to avoid that is to focus on my <u>own</u> health and not care what other people are doing or saying. Especially with my clients because they will say a lot of crazy things and the best response for me is to smile and nod in agreement because it might be working for them. My basic position is exactly that— figure it out for <u>yourself</u>.

That's what I did
FOR ME. So if I'm
59 years old and taking
no medications and
haven't had a medical exam
for over fifteen years,
I don't tell other people
to do that. It's what
I did. My best learnings
I first RESISTED, so I know
other people will resist
what I might explain, or
recommend, and that's
part of the process.
There's quite a vast
spectrum

of what people are doing for their health and on one end they might look at what I do and say, "you are so _extremist_," while at the other end say, "What a sell-out." I incorporate that into my model for what I suggest to clients and that is — make your own choices and offer no apology. (Inconsistency is to be expected.)

My approach to intestinal parasites might be expressed by an analogy. It's like I went

to Mt. Rushmore in
South Dakota and somebody
asks me what I see.
"I see a mountain," I
reply. So I go back the
next year and somebody
asks me what I see." I
see a mountain." They
ask: "Do you see any
faces?"
    I reply: "No, I
only see a mountain."
    This happens every
year for 15 years.
    Every year it is the
        same.

The sixteenth year,
I visit Mt. Rushmore
with a friend. They ask
me what I see. I say:
"I see a mountain."
They ask: "Can you
see a <u>nose?</u>"
I reply: "Barely,
maybe."
Suddenly, the whole
image falls into place.
What do I say?
"OMG! I was blind!"

Sometimes that's just how it works. I don't care how many people would have insisted right in my face that Americans could likely be widespread inhabited by parasitic worms. I've had said, "Not seeing it."

Given my 180 degree turn of opinion, one might expect that I would be THRILLED that Dr. Oz devoted one of his shows to the topic.

The show's announcer
states: " More than
40 million Americans
have already been
infected with a parasite."
On the first take of hearing
this news, it's shocking.
Whhat?
Whhen?
Where??
How?!
Wait a minute! "40 million"
is a statistical number and
we want to know who
counted and how did
they count?

There's just no way anybody could know. If the Dr. Oz show stated "There's 40 million rats living in New York City," there's not a way to **count** that either, nor verify. This statistic is quoted within the first 90 seconds, which tells us there's **two levels** to the coming message. Dr. Oz is winking to any viewer who has taken college math—"this show is not for you" because we've already signaled that the show is twisting statistics with impossibility. What the television writers _are_ saying is that "we know our target demographic is THE GULLIBLE and ratings _matter_ because this is HOLLYWOOD."

Later in the show, Dr. Oz suggests to "eat two cloves of garlic every day." This is actually excellent advice, which is covered for about one minute on the show.

<u>BUT</u> <u>Two</u> <u>cloves</u> is **not** a dosage. If you've ever pulled apart a garlic bulb, you would know that clove <u>size</u> varies greatly. Two large cloves could be equal to ten small cloves and if you are eating it raw, as they suggest, two large cloves is **WAY** too much. If you have ever eaten raw garlic cloves, this is THE <u>FIRST</u> <u>thing</u> you would point out because

in this case, size matters. The beneficial quality of raw garlic must be **chewed** to be released and activated. The average mortal human being would not be able to tolerate chewing a _medium_ sized garlic clove without something to cut the intensity such as honey or a huge spoon of ice cream. The other major problem is that raw garlic on an empty stomach will trigger an instant **gag** reflex and you will stand there overcome by the feeling you will **vomit.**

One of **Dr. Oz**'s hallmarks is that he tries lots of crazy stuff himself on the show, but he's not going to demonstrate <u>chewing</u> <u>raw</u> <u>garlic</u> for the audience because if he did, yes, he will be incapacitated for a good several minutes.

He tells us that eating garlic "will relax you." Whhhat? He says it will "keep people away from you." His guest doctor says, "This is terrible for your love life."

They recommend it, but not <u>seriously</u>.

When Dr. Oz sips the
wormwood tea, he says,
"This ... could <u>kill</u>
things!"
The audience laughs
and breaks into applause.
Yeah it's a funny moment,
but I don't think that
"a doctor going on television"
to tell people to do something
<u>he has never tried</u> is
something to clap over.
The featured guest
hasn't ever tasted it
either because she says,
"wwoo!"

So there's _two levels_, and the one level is for the gullible, which is to "do what I say, not what I do." Dr. Oz is likewise telling us— "Hey, I'm not doing any of this. This show is for **ratings** only."

The last "_easy_ parasite prevention" Dr. Oz _RECOMMENDATION_ is to consume half a cup of papaya seeds with one tablespoon of honey for "about ten days in a row," and

of all the recommendations,
this is the <u>best one</u>, they said.
They can't really be serious,
so there <u>HAS</u> <u>GOT</u> to be
a different message or
objective. It's obvious that
neither Dr. OZ nor his expert
gastroenterologist guest has
<u>tried this at home</u>. Papaya
seeds when dried are a
substitute for <u>peppercorns</u>.
Chewing <u>one</u> is almost too
much SPICE. Ten will throw
you into a serious GAG.
They say to eat
<u>half a cup</u>. (Oy!)

I had to replay the video 3X to believe that their suggestion is "half a cup of seeds" to one tablespoon of honey. The gastroenterologist then stated that "75% of children infected with parasites got results from doing this. I'm sorry, but no child, I or adult know is going to down 1/2 | cup of something like peppercorns daily for 10 days no matter how much honey you offer them.

My take on Dr. Oz's parasite exposé, is that the show was <u>INTENDED</u> as a joke.

Dr. Oz asks his doctor-guest the SOURCE of all these parasite infestations — and the answer was — contaminated water. The example given was Milwaukee, where 400,000 residents acquired parasitic illness via their TAP WATER. Later, Dr. Oz asks how the viewer audience can block parasite infection and the answer is to WASH YOUR HANDS.

I would assume that the doctor means with TAP WATER?

Plus, she suggests—
wash all fruits and
vegetables because many
of these are grown in <u>foreign
countries</u> with poor
sanitation standards,
but I think what she meant
was, **unless** you live in
Milwaukee. If she just
stated that the #1 source
of parasite infestation is
WATER, wouldn't washing
your fruit with water
<u>give</u> you parasites?
So it's a joke. It's the
kind of joke where Dr. Oz
can hang out with his doctor
friends and they can

tell him — "GREAT
show on 'PARASITES,'
Dr. OZ!"
      wink,
         wink. "slap on the"
                    back.
(we loved the total
      nonsense!)
and then Dr. OZ can
say, "Who'd like
some Wormwood tea?"

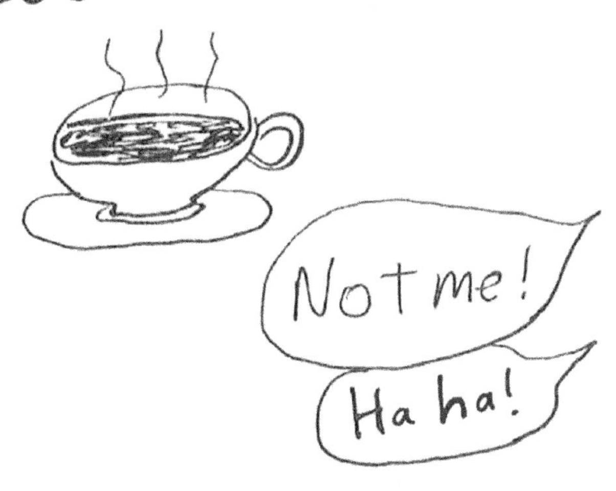

# Chapter 2

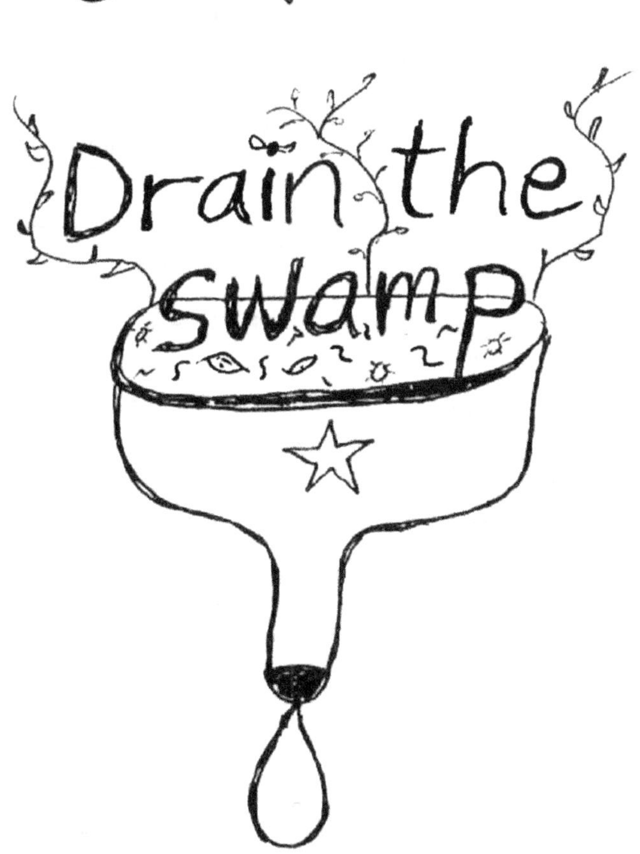

When you're in school,
whether high school or
college, much of what
we learn is just the
broad strokes.

Much of what we
did learn will soon be
outdated and maybe later
even proven incorrect.

The topic of
parasites in terms of
a collected **BODY** of
**knowledge** I'd guess
is somewhere between
preschool and
kindergarten $\longrightarrow$

in its development.
I would expect that
most anybody with a Ph.D.
in parasitology would
be the first to agree
that we _don't_ _know_ _much_
about it. If you go on
YouTube and watch a few
films of people talking
about parasites or parasite
cleanses, you can bet
that they don't know much
about it. If you bring
up the topic with your
chiropractor, your acupuncturist,
your health guru of

Whatever persuasion or your average M.D., they won't know much about it. The next time you see your doctor, ask them to tell you what they know about human parasites. Do they deflect the question? Set a stopwatch. How much time do they give you to educate you on the topic? Now I might be spending lots of time exploring it, but most doctors would say that **I'm** the hack.

My whole thing is
centered on one thing—
what I've seen with
my <u>own</u> <u>eyes</u>.
A friend of mine
who works at Vanderbilt
Hospital said a patient
was brought to the emergency
room with an open gut
wound after a car accident
and there were large
worms crawling out.
Now if a doctor working there
just received a Ph.D. in
parasitology, nobody will
talk about it. <u>Seeing</u>
worms — totally different!

I doubt there's more than a dozen colon hygienists across the state of Tennessee where I live. I'd guess that 99% of Americans have never received a colonic and probably 99.9% of doctors have not. But there are lots of opinions!

I'd probably administered 12,000 colonics before I realized I had been looking at worms and not seeing them.

A significant aspect
to note is that the
flora and fauna showing
their faces are DEAD.
What if all the birds we
ever saw were two days
dead? Or eaten by a fox
and passed through its gut?
We couldn't imagine how
birds could sing, build
nests or dart through a
tree. A dead bird is
nothing like a living
bird. Most parasites I
see in the colonic water —
it doesn't resemble them in
their natural habitat.

Now I have captured
what I consider AMAZING
photos of wormy things
coming out in the colonic
water, but how I'd describe
what I mostly <u>see</u> appears
as if somebody took a fish
bait bucket of <u>crawdads</u>,
<u>leeches</u> and <u>minnows</u>,
put it in a blender and
ran it for two seconds,
let it sit in the hot sun
all day, and that's the
sort of detritus making
its exit through the
colonic tubing.

on the other hand,
There's a <u>YouTube</u> video
filming a technician
catching a parasitic fluke
living inside a person.
A cable with a tweezer-
like instrument has a grip
on this fluke and it's putting
up a _fight_ like a swordfish.
A fluke looks like a two-inch
stingray and this film
shows it <u>kicking</u> and <u>screaming</u>
and dragging its feet,
fully against its own will.
So if you had a fluke
in your body, you can see,
getting it to leave
wouldn't be **easy**.

Now I consider myself to be a world authority on health, which happened somewhat accidentally and resulting from my own curiosity. I remember back in college taking a difficult philosophy course and finding myself totally lost. It was like this:

One of my friends in the class was particularly adept at grasping the <u>BIG picture</u>. So I'd ask him about it and he'd nonchalantly explain it in about a paragraph's worth of conversation, I'd get the missing piece, and the whole thing would fall into place.

A few years ago, I realized that this was the same with health care.

Plus I recognized that **_LEVERAGE_** is critical because I've talked to THOUSANDS of people about their health and MOST expend a huge amount of energy doing things for their health which have almost **nothing** related to their <u>core health</u> <u>concerns.</u>

One thing I know for certain, after administering 12,000 colonics, is that the demographics of my clients are all over the board and represent a random sample of the U.S. population. 100% of their colons have been <u>full</u> of fecal matter.

What doctors tell us is that the human body naturally self cleanses with a normal American healthy diet.

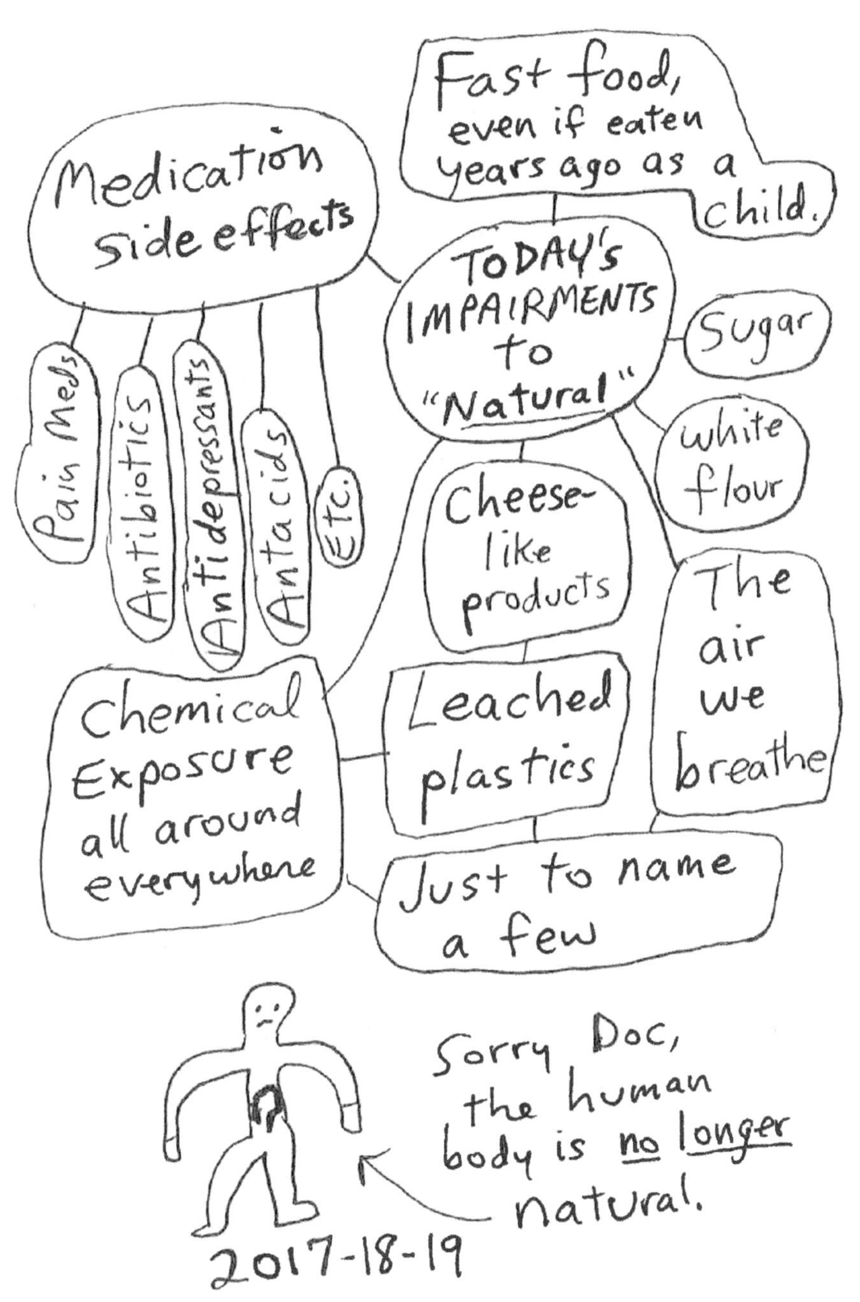

Medication side effects
Fast food, even if eaten years ago as a child.
TODAY'S IMPAIRMENTS to "Natural"
Sugar
white flour
Pain Meds
Antibiotics
Antidepressants
Antacids
Etc.
Cheese-like products
The air we breathe
Chemical Exposure all around everywhere
Leached plastics
Just to name a few
Sorry Doc, the human body is no longer natural.
2017-18-19

It seems to me, that
doctors tend to oversimplify
what colon hygienists do
and say:

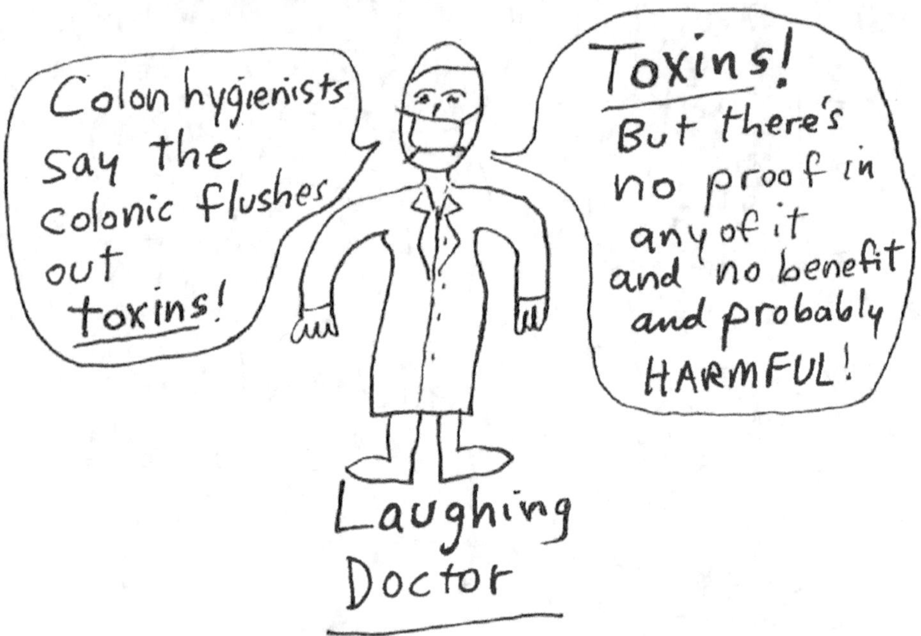


As a stand-alone term,
I would agree, "toxin"
has almost no meaning.
To say, "The body builds up
toxins'" is equally nebulous.

What's actually going on, if doctors actually had a conversation with a few colon hygienists, is that colon hygienists SEE a <u>certain</u> something and know they function as a feedback loop in society.

The human body eliminates naturally — Base Truth

Other conclusions drawn

Medical Paradigm

If a colon hygienist is a **feedback loop** suggesting that Americans might NO LONGER be eliminating naturally, that would perhaps shift the medical paradigm in the drive to understand people increasingly <u>ill</u> from mystery illnesses.

And IF Americans over the past four or five or six decades have been losing function in the internal organs, and not just the colon, then colon hygienists might be the <u>first</u> social feedback loop to notice.

What I did was to start MAPPING OUT what colon hygienists were seeing. I read a news headline which said: DEPRESSION DISCOVERED TO CAUSE OSTEOPOROSIS!

From a colon hygienist's perspective, this would be a misreading of the data.

So I mapped out a simple flow chart, working backwards.

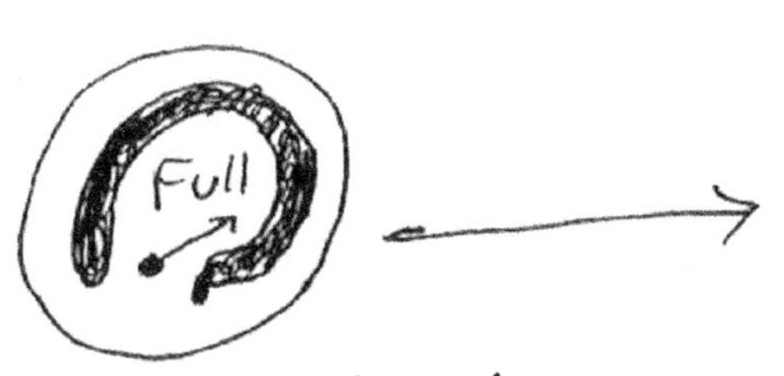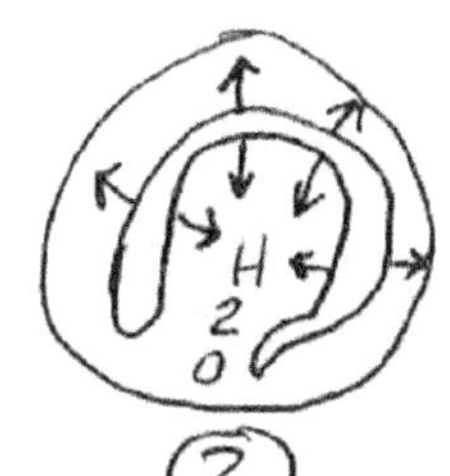


① In recent decades, most American's cOlons are abnormally full.

② One JoB the Colon does is to extract water from the feces.

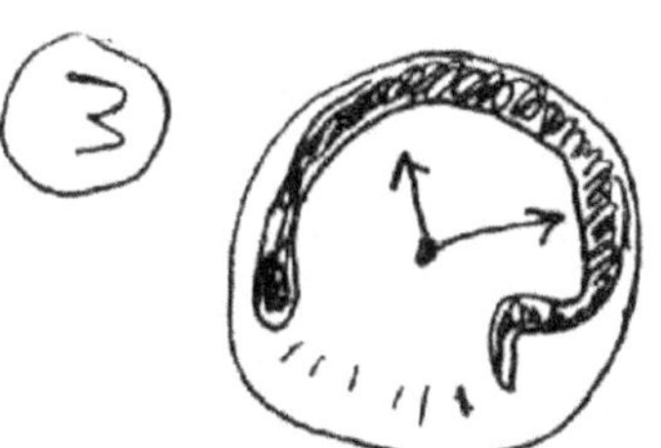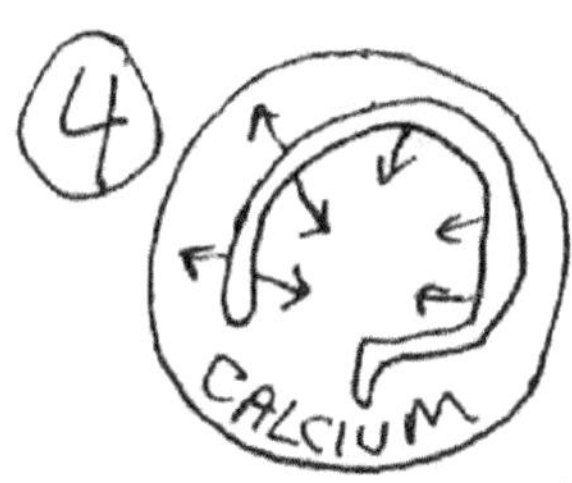


③ A FULL cOlon slows transit time.

④ Calcium is absorbed through theColon wall into the blood.

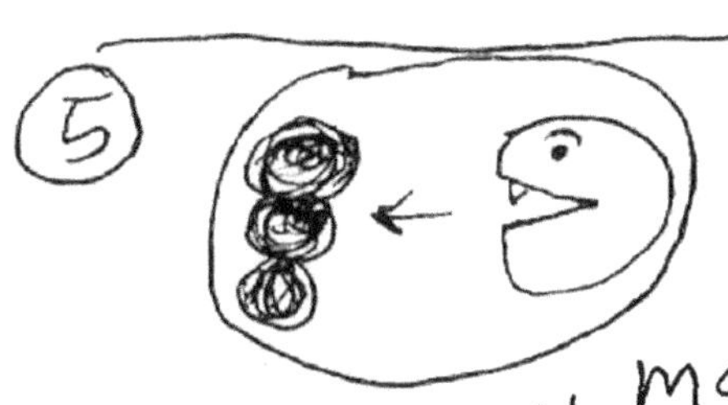

⑤ Bacteria living inside the colon consume fecal matter which makes the calcium bio-available.

(6) 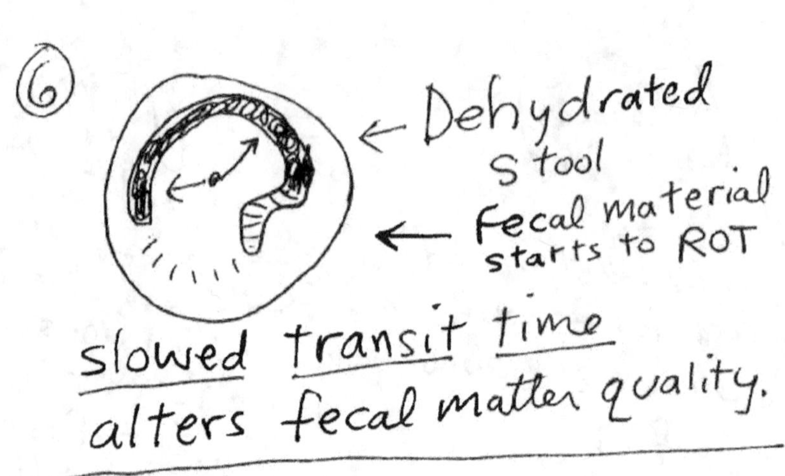


<u>slowed transit time</u> alters fecal matter quality.

(7)

Rotten, dry fecal matter feeds the wrong types of bacteria and fungi, causing them to proliferate.

(8) These non-beneficial bacteria & fungi are ALIVE, creating their own <u>wastes</u> in the colon, which are slightly toxic to the human host.

9. 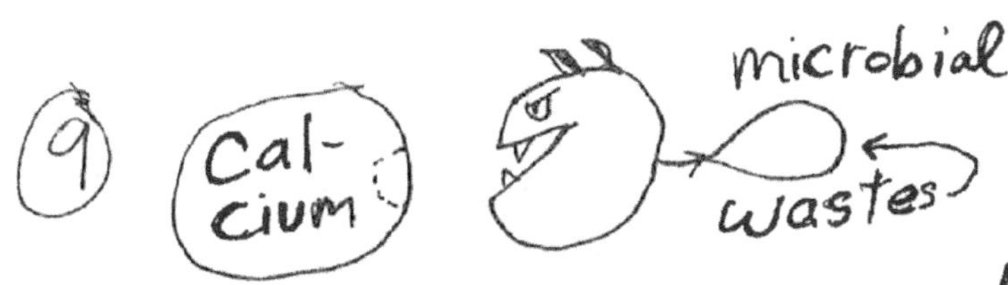


As calcium is consumed and released in this negative environment, it is less bio-available for absorption into the blood.

10. 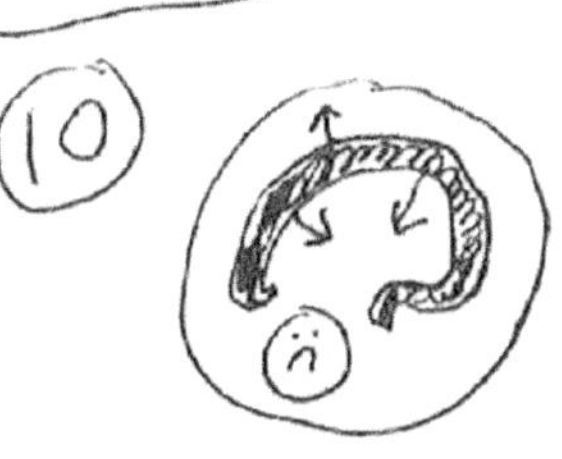
Calcium is important for many bodily functions, including balancing blood pH.

11. To prevent ACIDITY, the bones leach stored calcium FROM the bones, which over time contributes to osteoporosis.

12. Plus, these harmful bacterial wastes enter the blood, like ammonia + methanes, causing depression.

⑬ But the situation is actually <u>worse</u> than that.

⑭ 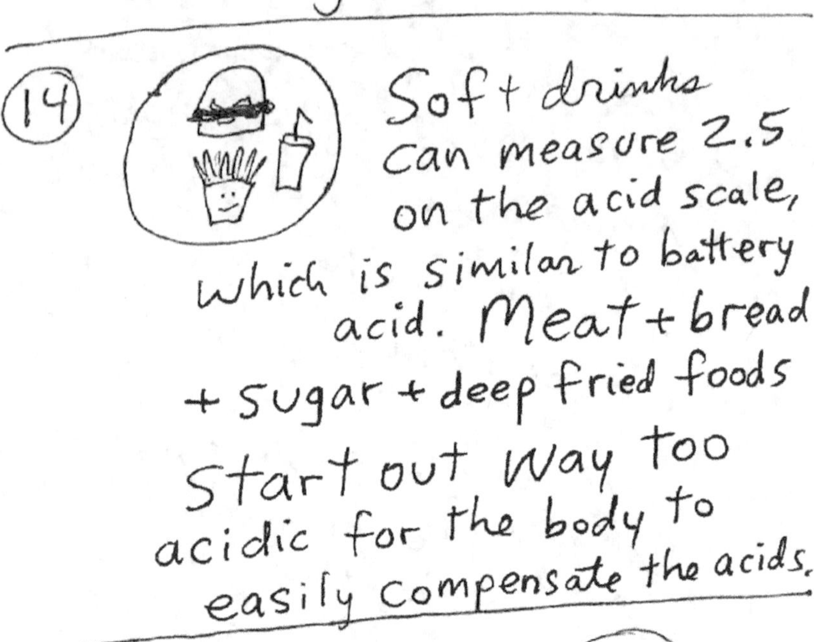
Soft drinks can measure 2.5 on the acid scale, which is similar to battery acid. Meat + bread + sugar + deep fried foods start out way too acidic for the body to easily compensate the acids.

⑮ Therefore, <u>MORE</u> calcium leaches from the bones.

⑯ 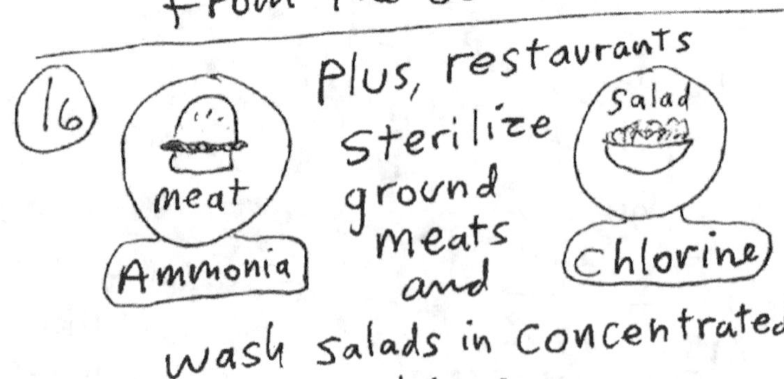

Plus, restaurants sterilize ground meats and wash salads in concentrated chlorine.

(17) So this triggers harmful problems at the FRONT END of digestion too, which further impairs what happens in the Colon.

---

(18) The Sterilizing agents and anti-biotic additives continue to Kill bacteria inside the human, including in the small intestine.

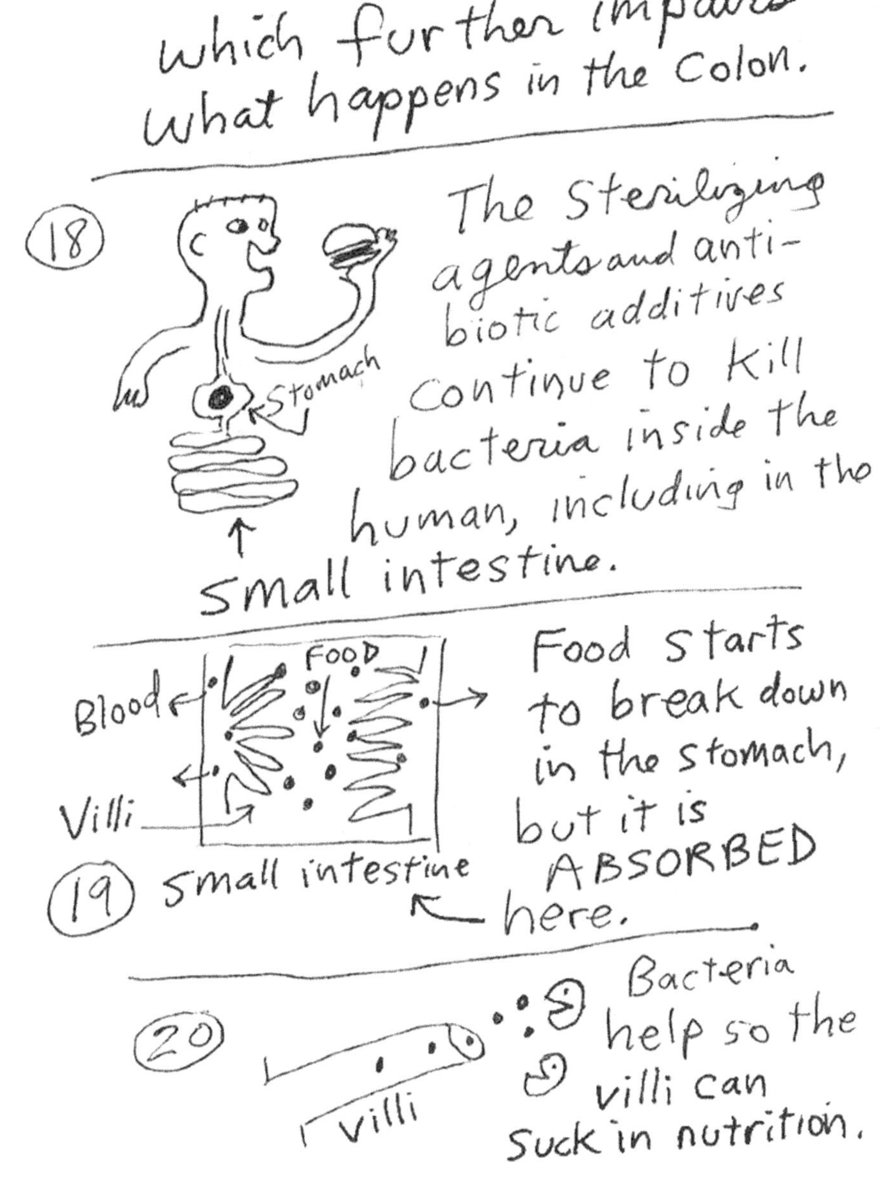


---

Food starts to break down in the stomach, but it is ABSORBED here.

(19) 

---

(20) Bacteria help so the villi can suck in nutrition.



153

(21)



These small intestinal bacteria are called "acidophilus" because their waste is ACIDIC, because here acids HELP iron to be bio-available so the villi can pass iron into the blood.

(22) But if there are sterilizing agents in the FOOD, this kills the acidophilus.

(23)



So the iron molecules can't get into the blood, plus the iron will help to make poop harden in the colon.

(24) Plus the villi straws will suck up the antibiotics and send it to the human's liver, where it will further kill beneficial bacteria there.



(25) Now the liver is more toxic. The liver de-toxifies the blood, but without beneficial bacteria, what will detoxify the liver?

(26)



155

27.) The human liver begins to _store_ the molecules of these chemicals. These resist water, so the liver loses moisture.

28 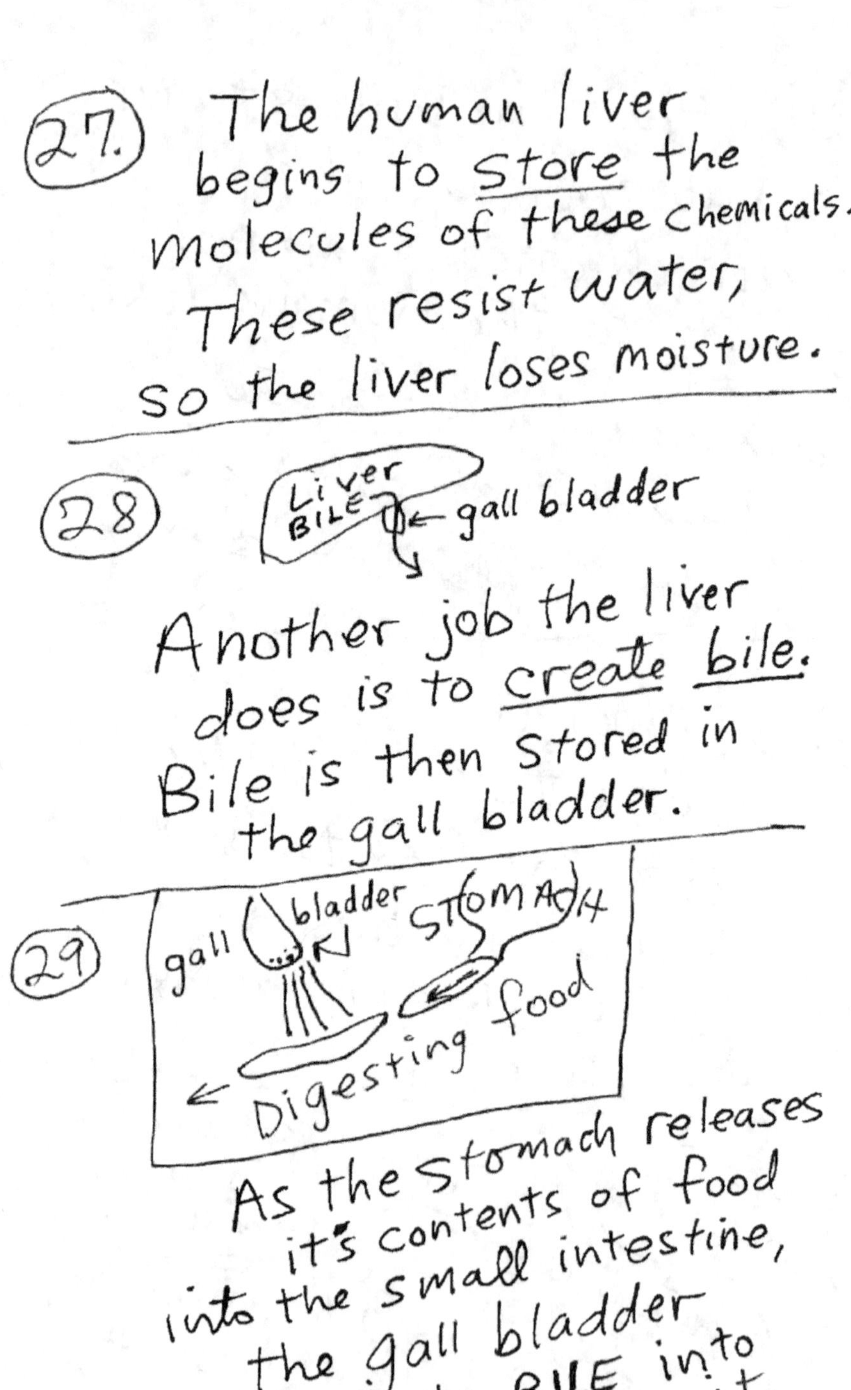


Another job the liver does is to _create_ _bile_. Bile is then stored in the gall bladder.

29 As the stomach releases it's contents of food into the small intestine, the gall bladder squirts _BILE_ into it.

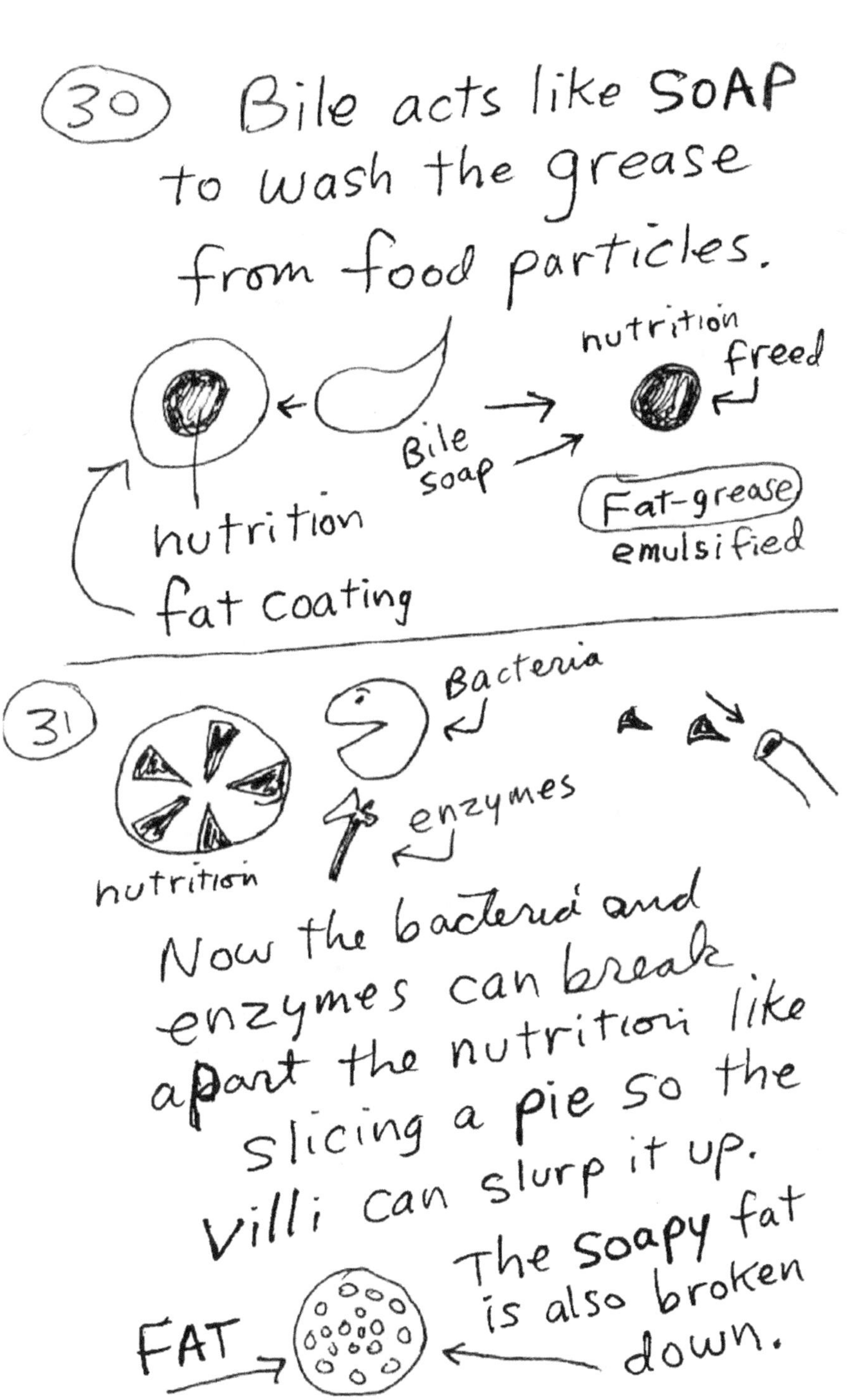

30 Bile acts like SOAP to wash the grease from food particles.
nutrition
freed
Bile soap
Fat-grease emulsified
nutrition
fat coating
31
Bacteria
nutrition
enzymes
Now the bacteria and enzymes can break apart the nutrition like slicing a pie so the villi can slurp it up.
The soapy fat is also broken down.
FAT

(32)



But a dry and exhausted liver produces less bile, and with less bile soap to go around, some of the nutrition remains coated by fat.



(33) This inhibits nutrient absorption and fat assimilation.

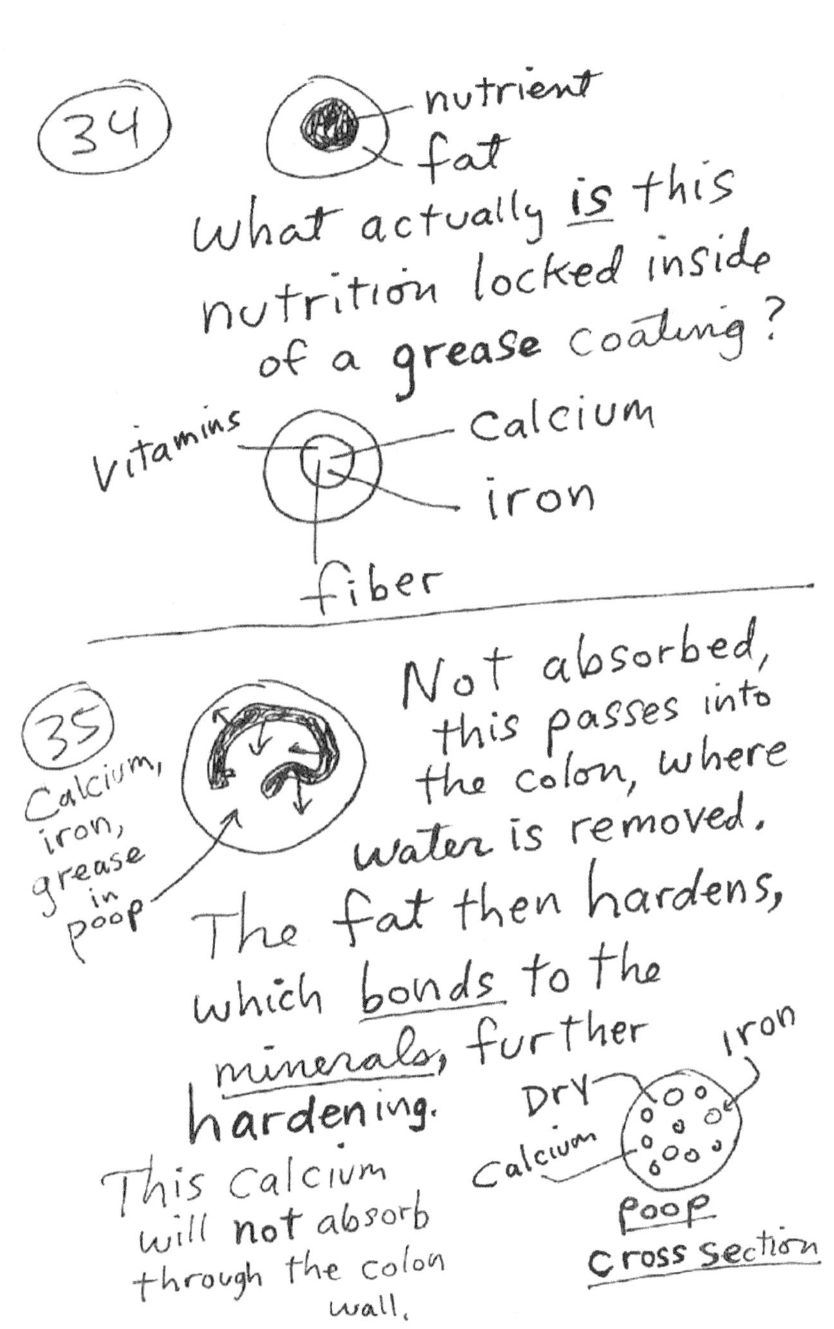
34
nutrient
fat
What actually _is_ this nutrition locked inside of a **grease** coating?
vitamins
Calcium
iron
fiber

35
Calcium, iron, grease in poop
Not absorbed, this passes into the colon, where water is removed. The fat then hardens, which _bonds_ to the _minerals_, further hardening.
This calcium will **not** absorb through the colon wall.
Dry
Calcium
iron
poop
cross section

(36) Meanwhile, back in the small intestine, bacterial <u>acids</u> have been preventing <u>yeasts from multiplying.</u>

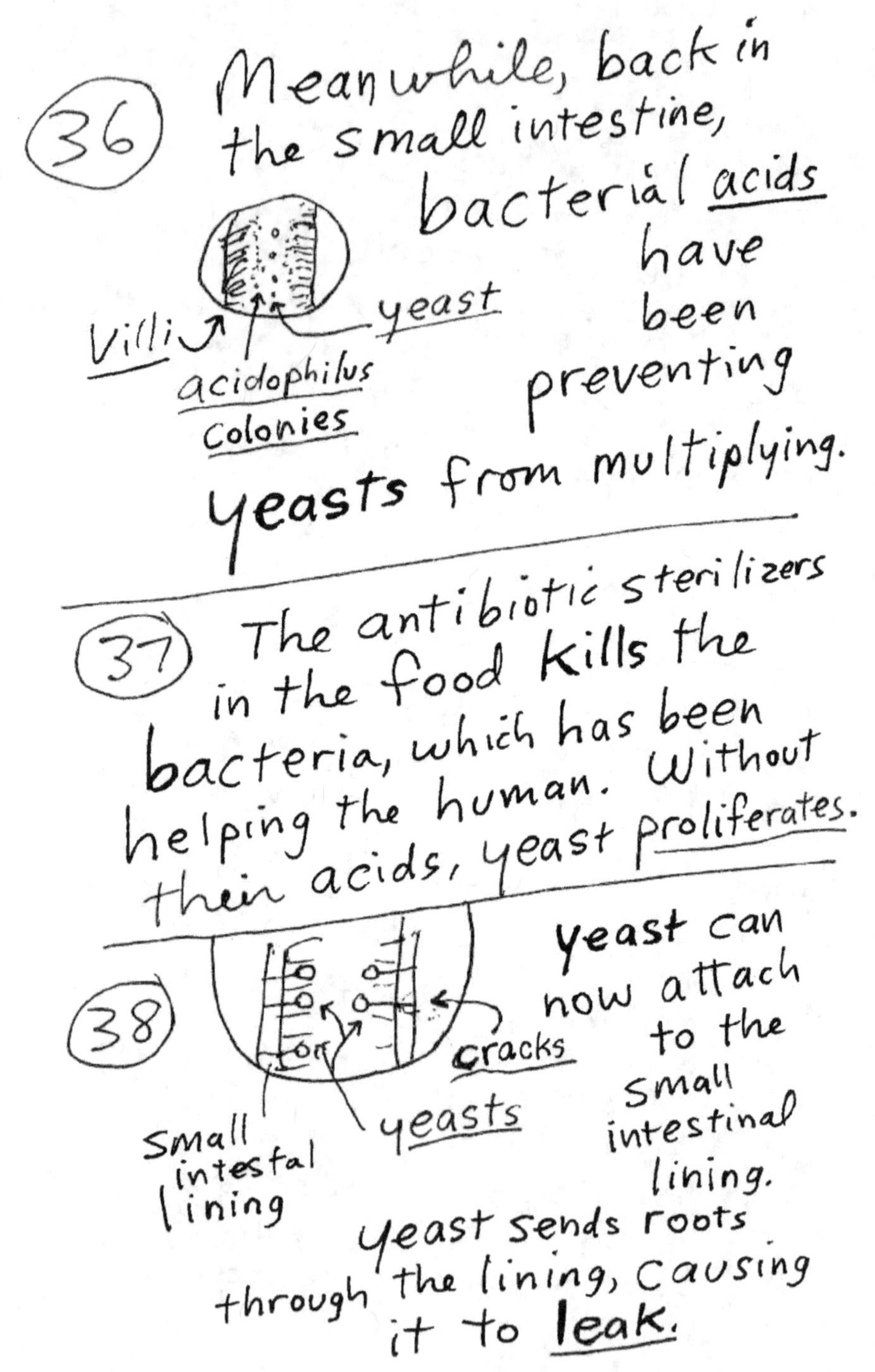


(37) The antibiotic sterilizers in the food kills the bacteria, which has been helping the human. Without their acids, <u>yeast proliferates.</u>

(38) yeast sends roots through the lining, causing it to <u>leak.</u>

(39) The body's natural line of protection has been **breached!**

(40) Undigested food particles start leaking into the human's blood, triggering an immune reaction to mop up this problem.

(41) Certain types of undigested food particles, like soy, wheat or peanuts, can trigger histamines and an allergic reaction.

(42) o — iron
o — sugar
o — oxygen
The yeast escapes into the blood too, scavenging critical iron and consuming sugar to grow and reproduce.

(43) plus the candida yeast itself is poisonous, like poison ivy, except really, really tiny.

(44) Now the blood is pumping through the liver, which is attempting to filter the candida out.

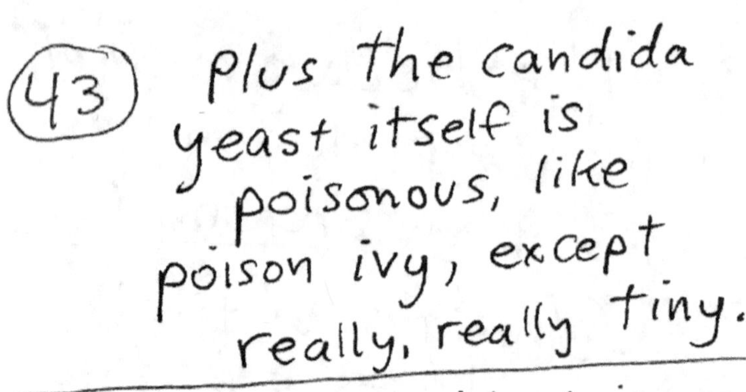



(45) This is a bit of a crisis, so the liver creates its own antifungal secretion called hesperin, but this inhibits communication between the liver and thyroid.
(T4 to T3)

(46) Now basic metabolism can't properly regulate. Stomach acidity declines which reduces vitamin B·12 production and energy starts to crash.

(47) Sugar craving increases to meet energy needs, which the body also converts to fat, due to low nutritional fat assimilation, due to reduced bile production. With toxicity in the liver and the blood, plus a growing sack of shit at the bottom end, this person is about to become even more **depressed.**

(48) Now the media comes out and reports some latest clinical study that "depression causes ~~an~~ osteoporosis."

No, this person was losing bone density long before depression set in.

---

(49) Then a doctor goes on television and <u>ridicules</u> colon hygienists, suggesting they tell people to do colonics to pull out "their toxins." No Doc, that's **not** what we say.

50.) What we might say
would be more like —

- The condition of the colon appears to be affected by the health of the liver.
- Because the liver is self-cleansing, positioned at the top of the intestines, if the colon itself has become congested with calcified poop, it might make sense to somehow pull all that out, so what the liver purges can actually **exit** the body.
- Water administered into

the colon might help
to <u>hydrate</u> a part
of the body which could
be on the <u>dry</u> side.
• A colon hygienist has
nothing against the dairy
industry, while they
themselves wouldn't suggest
drinking **milk** to "supplement
calcium" if the issue is
not calcium intake, but
<u>up</u>take. Plus, certain
foods can form into **mucus,**
which can get into the
colon and sandwich into
mucus layers, which when
dehydrated, harden into
glue which will <u>bond together</u>
several meals of food.

• Now if your drain was stopped up, you wouldn't hire a plumber and tell all your friends that when he walked through the door, he said he was there to get "your toxins out." No colon hygienist I know says to a client: "Thank God you're here so I can get your toxins out!" If we're doing anything, we are helping to undo what the rest of the world has unwittingly done to poison the human race.

# 3

# Paradigm

Many medical institutions, including Mayo Clinic, and medical advice television programs, including <u>The Doctors</u> and <u>Dr. Oz</u>, and most doctors, present a very different picture of what a colonic does:

Some people will suggest that doctors are against colonics because "doctors fear colonics will cut in on their business." This couldn't be further from the truth.

Medical expenses total **25%** of GNP.



What Americans spend on colonics annually isn't even a **pencil point** on the map. Plus, most doctors are trying their best to help their patients be healthy.

Doctors <u>truly</u> <u>believe</u> what they say about colonics! The only problem is they know nothing about it.



There could be multiple ill conditions and symptoms better explained and better treated if "backed-up colons" were better understood as SYSTEMIC and common, even afflicting medical experts and their families!

I wrote about this in great detail in my other books, <u>Inside Poop</u> and <u>The Conspiracy Theory Diet</u>. So I wouldn't want to repeat myself regarding my opinion that colonics are a perfect tool to unplug directly at the point where people are having trouble, whether they know it or **not**.

Many people's colons will actually bulge-out with excess poop.

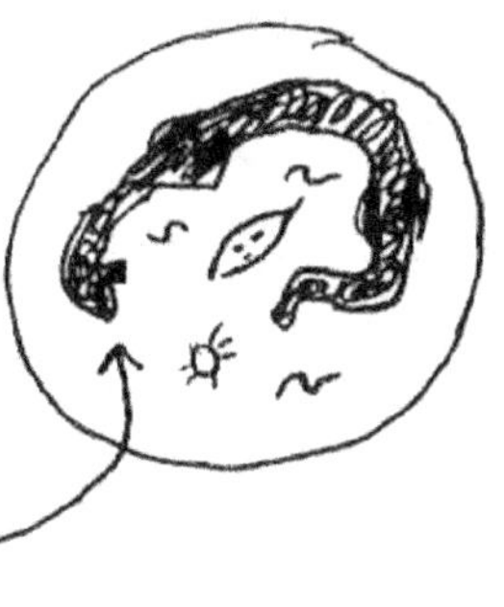

This creates the perfect breeding ground for larger parasites.

What we would look
for to support the
hypothesis that America's
colons have backed up,
are the statistics
measuring the rise or
fall of many common
diseases afflicting the
nation.

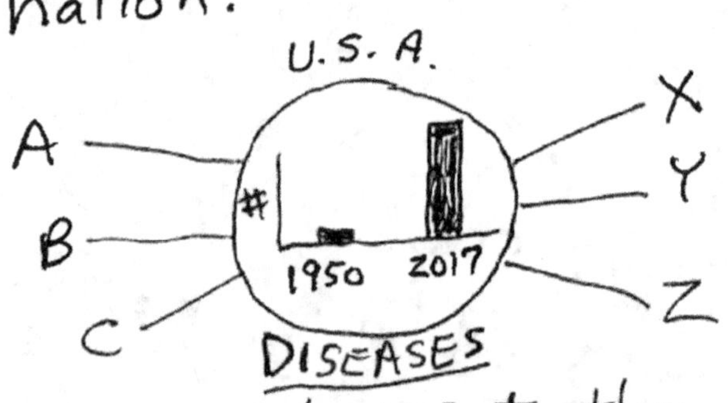


Maybe look into the
history of the illnesses
you or your loved ones
have been diagnosed
with because they have
mostly SKYROCKETED.

When I really got to thinking about it, I realized that I could reasonably PREDICT illnesses and help to prevent them if I put my understanding into a smart phone app. I mapped the whole thing. Then I took my maps down to Nashville's local entrepreneur center and met with an advisor consultant, who happened to be the former Dean at the Owen Business School at Vanderbilt, with a specialty expertise in health care.

Not very long into my presentation, he said:
"Where's your clinical studies ?!"
I explained that our current health care system model has been <u>based</u> <u>on</u> <u>clinical studies</u> and suggested that "clinical studies" are the <u>constraint</u> to progress. This is partially due to the fact that <u>PROBLEM</u> Ⓐ is caused by <u>PROBLEM</u> Ⓑ which is caused by <u>PROBLEM</u> Ⓒ. And there is no way

Clinical studies can PROVE Problem Ⓒ, so you can't solve PROBLEM Ⓐ if you are depending on clinical studies to substantiate Problem Ⓒ. Plus, in some cases, Problem Ⓒ is CAUSED by the health care industry itself and we know that the health care industry does not like to point any fingers at itself.
This went straight over his head.

He replied: "If you are making <u>any kind</u> of <u>recommendations</u> without clinical studies, there's the broad possibility that <u>you</u> could <u>hurt</u> somebody."

I politely countered: "You are well aware that you make that statement within the context that our current system, <u>based</u> on clinical studies, is HURTING thousands of Americans <u>every day</u>. By its own admission, the pharmaceutical industry is killing at minimum 10,000 Americans per MONTH and this is not due to the fact that killing that many people is the other side to helping a bunch of other people. 'Medical error' is the fourth leading cause of death in this country and that doesn't include some of the lesser evils like paralysis or seizures or organ failures or RASHES for that matter, so **WHY NOT** see that a breakthrough could come from somebody like me?"

I knew what he was going to say as he started shaking his head: "You've got no proof and with no proof, you've got nothing."

I replied: "Oh but I do have proof!"

"WHERE is it?" he asked.

"My methodology is to string together truth statements in a new order," I explained. "Plus, _I'm_ proof! For my age and demographic, I've spent zero on medical costs the past 15 years, which is WAY outside the norm. more amazing

→

is that I know WHY, AND I can _duplicate_ my success. And if you took just a moment to look over what I've invented, not only would you see that nobody could be **hurt** by it, but you yourself might benefit because I think you would." I said earnestly.

Here's the thing: I didn't go down there to <u>argue</u> with anybody. For me, it's just a learning, talking to <u>him</u>.

What I learned was
this:

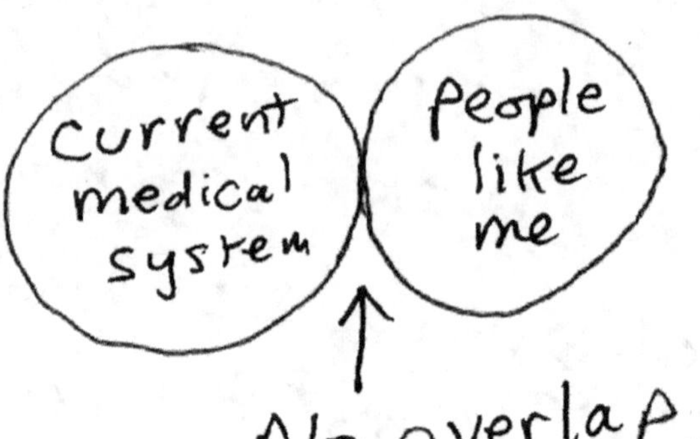


And then, there's him :

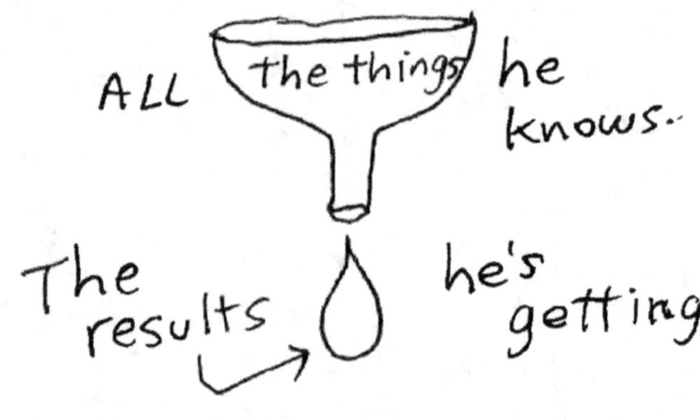


For him, there's **no**
**gap** in "what he knows,"
no "one thing" he _doesn't_
_know_, that he is anxious
to discover.

So I can respect this man,
that he set out to
accomplish certain things
in life and succeeded.
There's a certain <u>game</u> to
it and <u>he's</u> playing one
game and <u>I'm</u> playing
another. He's dressed to
play golf and I show up
with a tennis racquet.
And I know that! I knew
it first shaking his hand.
He's playing golf and
they're **ALL** playing <u>golf</u>.
He's not going to play <u>my</u>
game and I'm not
playing theirs.

# CHAPTER 4

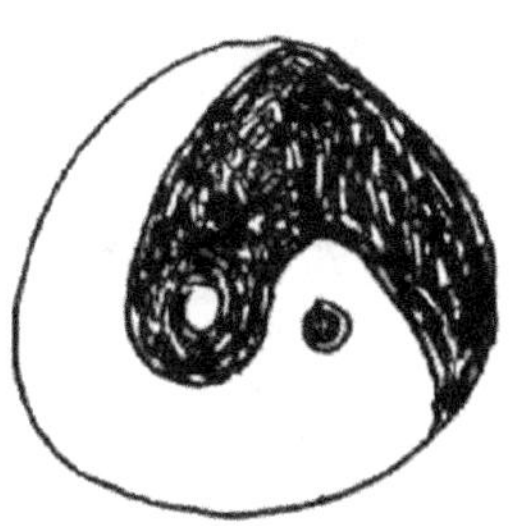

# Para·doxical

What I find fascinating about the medical field is that it sometimes makes its profits from nothing. For example, imagine a small _farming village_ where everybody has a job to do, which requires them to wake up at dawn, and all day long everybody works, works, works, such that not long after sunset, most everyone is _asleep_. What this village mainly produces is grains, fruits and vegetables.

A new stranger moves to town and opens a shop selling <u>sleeping pills</u>. The problem is, people from the village are having no trouble falling asleep.

When you are getting something for free, it's nothing anybody would pay for.

At the time of the birth of America and George Washington, health insurance hadn't been invented because there was no need for it.

Doctors at that time were kept busy by various emergencies and very little was addressed that wasn't rooted in practicality. Often, doctoring was a side-job to something else, like being the town undertaker or barber. It stayed pretty much like this for many decades. Even in 1960, the average American citizen was spending less than $15 per month on medical expenditures and nobody then would have predicted the outrageous health care issues or complexity of today.

what happened in 1960 to trigger a kind of revolution in doctoring was the introduction of the birth <u>control pill</u>. It was launched with great <u>skepticism</u> that anybody would BUY it.

But they did!

Now when somebody gets rich overnight, that's like a GOLD RUSH. Everybody starts showing up with a pick and a shovel. Every <u>bodily function</u> was suddenly game for <u>mining</u> like a bubbling crude.

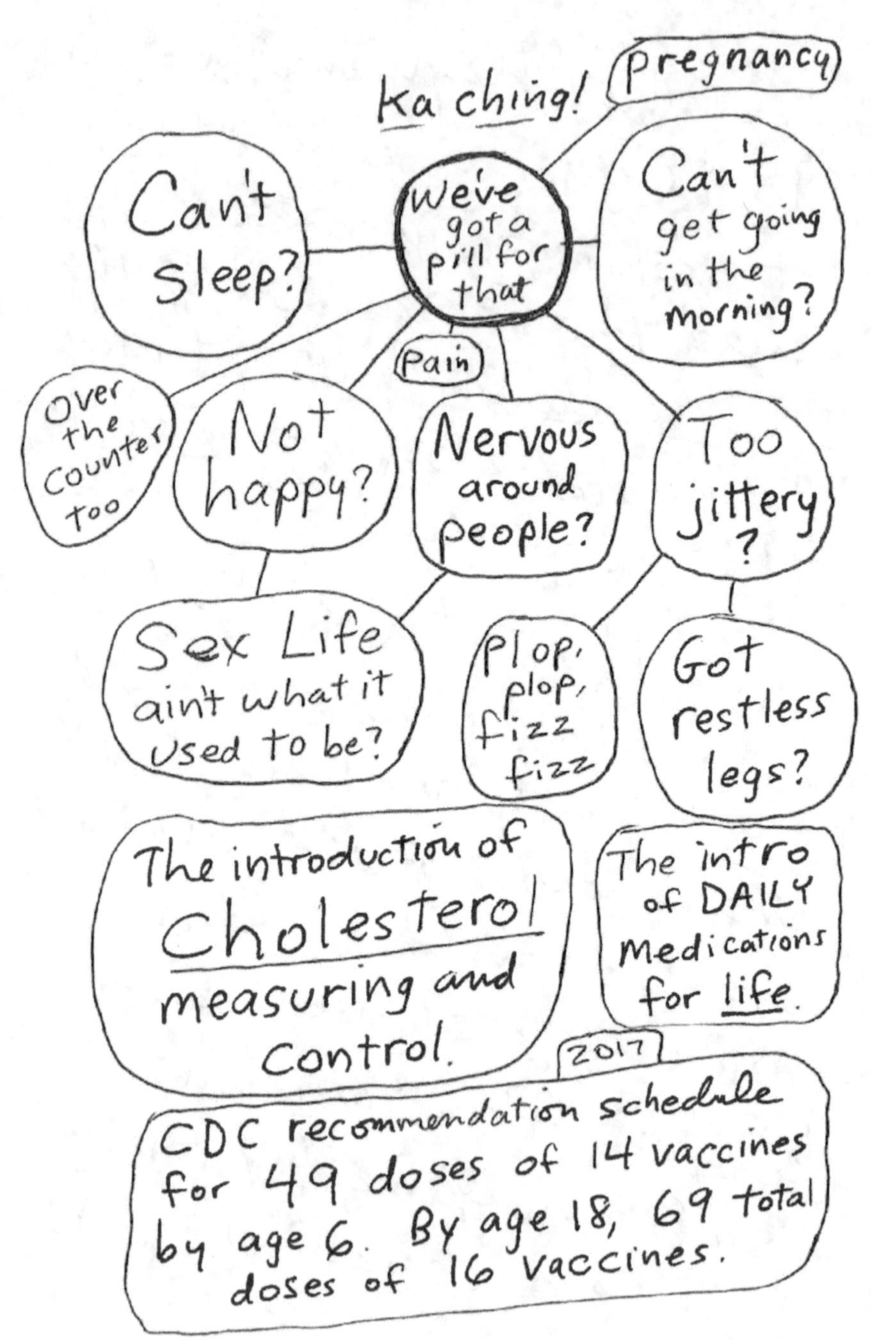
ka ching!
Pregnancy
Can't sleep?
We've got a pill for that
Can't get going in the morning?
Over the counter too
Pain
Not happy?
Nervous around people?
Too jittery?
Sex Life ain't what it used to be?
Plop, plop, fizz fizz
Got restless legs?
The introduction of Cholesterol measuring and control.
The intro of DAILY Medications for life.
2017
CDC recommendation schedule for 49 doses of 14 vaccines by age 6. By age 18, 69 total doses of 16 vaccines.

Then what you get
are _side effects_:

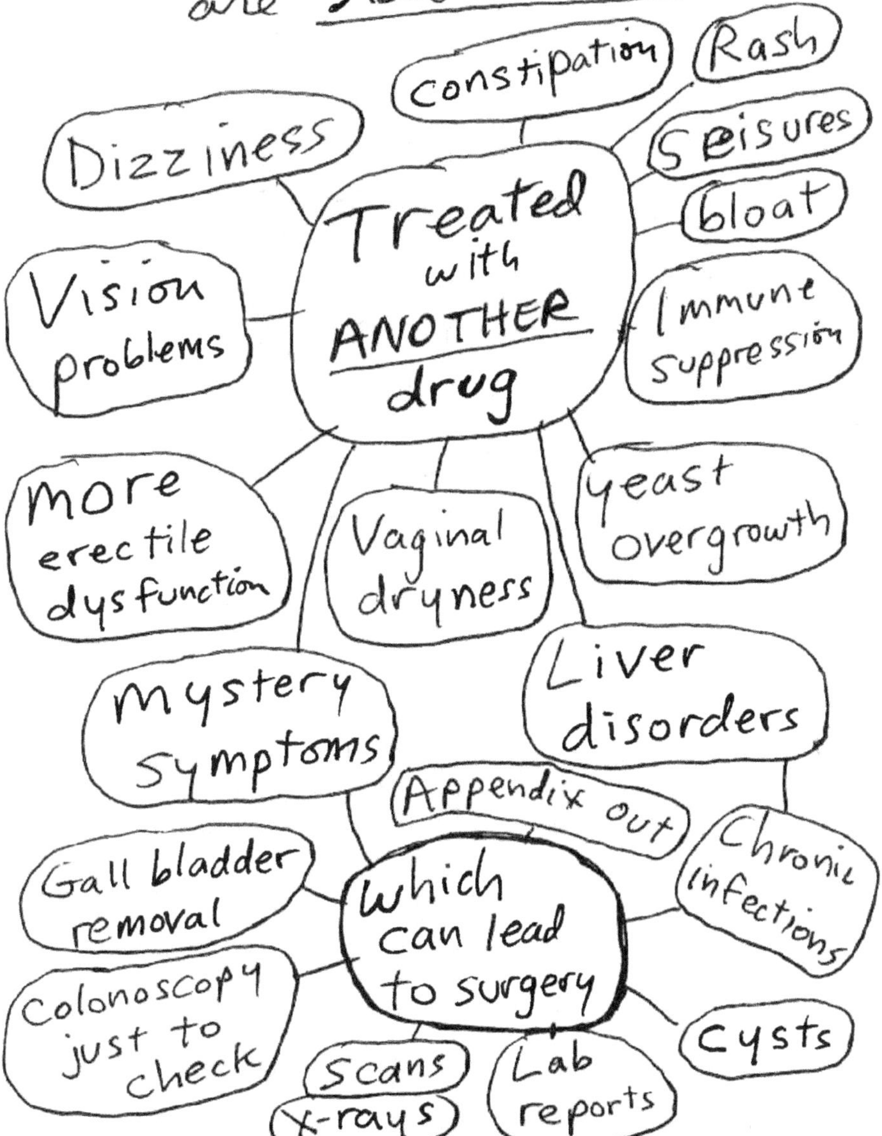

Constipation
Rash
Dizziness
Seisures
Treated with ANOTHER drug
bloat
Vision problems
Immune suppression
more erectile dysfunction
Vaginal dryness
yeast overgrowth
Liver disorders
mystery symptoms
Appendix out
Chronic infections
Gall bladder removal
which can lead to surgery
Colonoscopy just to check
Scans
X-rays
Lab reports
Cysts

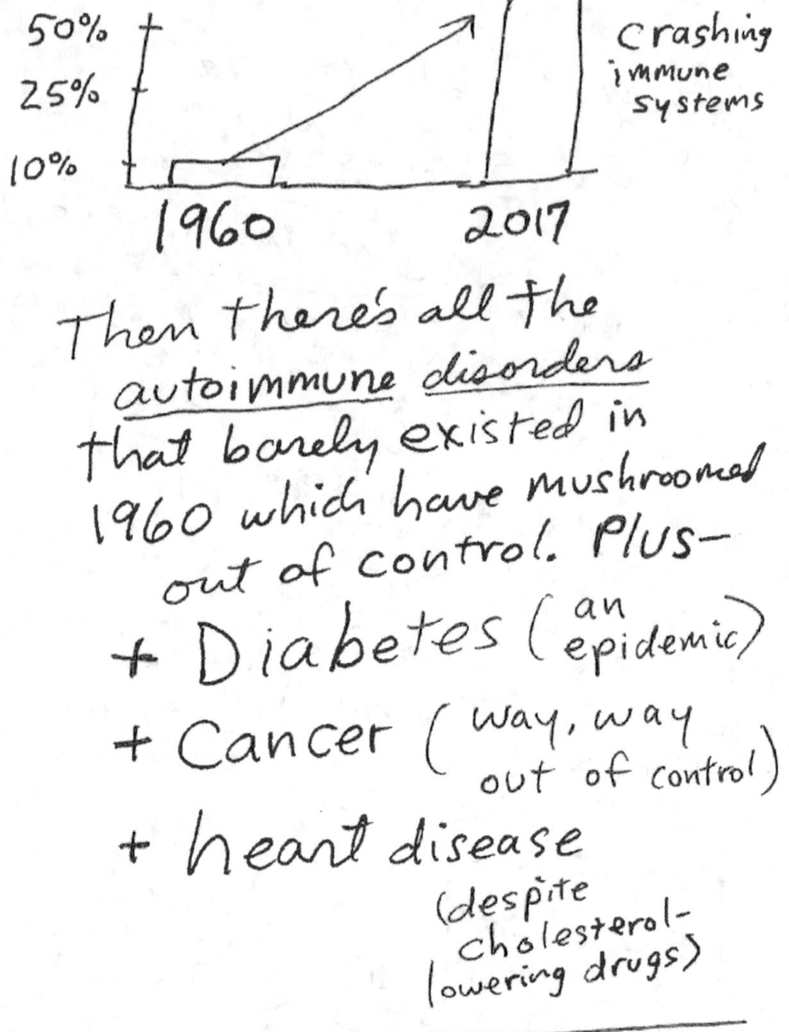



Then there's all the _autoimmune disorders_ that barely existed in 1960 which have mushroomed out of control. Plus—

+ Diabetes (an epidemic)

+ Cancer (way, way out of control)

+ heart disease (despite cholesterol-lowering drugs)

---

Realize that I really do remain _upbeat_ even if I invent a way to help the medical side of things and I am told to go home because I might hurt somebody.

what's interesting to me, you know, as somebody who has spent quite a bit of time studying philosophy and religion, is the space parasites hold within the human **psyche**. The average person doesn't want to think about it, not just because we have enough to think about, but what are the implications? And ramifications!

At the end of Stanley Kubrick's <u>2001: A Space Odyssey</u>, we observe a space child in a cosmic star

rebirth floating in space
inside of a shining placenta
of light, gazing upon Earth
as in wonder for the
potential it holds. What
stands out is the _sense_
of _intelligence_, cleanliness,
purity, that _consciousness_
_itself_ is the _ultimate_. But
the film is ruined if the
camera pans back from
the star child to reveal
the umbilical chord reaching

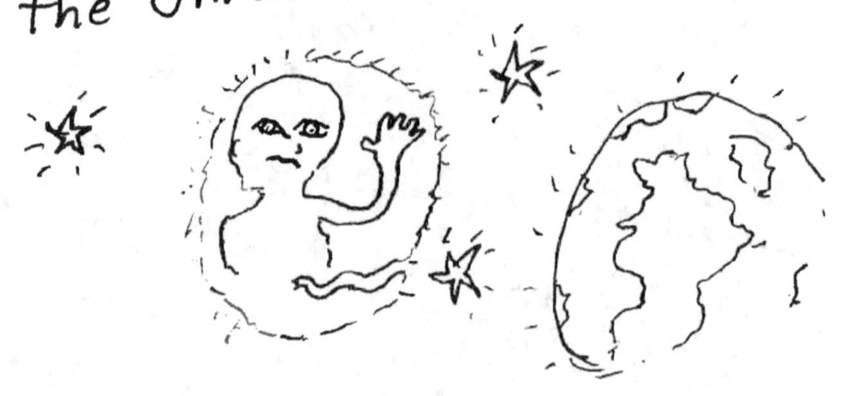

outwards is actually
a tapeworm.
Oh oh!
We are not alone!
And which is the
higher intelligence?
The Star Child withers
as the worm sucks out
its precious life force.
Now the worm detaches
and floats back towards
Earth.
God forbid!
It's a race and
now we must

have our Listerine,
our hand sanitizers and
disinfectant sprays, the
triple antibiotic lotions,
our skin slathered in protective
sunscreens and bug repellant
layers. We prefer our
root vegetables sprayed with
lab-inspired chemical inventions
to stop their sprouting,
then sliced into finger food
that's been deep fried in
scalding hot oil, salted and
served in a cardboard box.

I am well aware that the average reader is ready to get on with it, skim through the PROOF that Americans are commonly infected with VISIBLE parasites and 1) either laugh it off or 2) take a pill, sleep through the holocaust, then arise in the morning A-OK. If you have read this far, then I'm going to ask for another favor: Put your thinking cap back on.

I myself already know beyond the shadow of a doubt that the entire human race is infested with internal insect-like critters of multiple variety, many of which haven't been mapped. If rolled into a solid ball, the size of their mass in one individual could choke a horse. Stand on the scale to weigh yourself and how much do the internal parasites weigh? <u>Pounds</u>, not ounces. (2 lbs. wet, nothing dry.)

I'm just slightly ahead
of you with the revelation
of this and have already
suffered through the
emotional repercussions.
I've transversed this
dark alley multiple times
and have seen where
the manhole covers are
missing. I'd rather be
safe than sorry. For me
to explain certain seemingly
irrelevant details is part
of it. If you want to
cut to the chase, go

on YouTube right now,
search under "parasite
cleanse," watch till your
eyes are red, attempt
a few lame protocols,
fail, then tell yourself
that it's Scott's fault.
This is not about
getting *your* *worms* out
in the next 10 minutes.
This is the point in the
movie where James Dean
hits his head against the
wall and says, "why,
why, why?"

If the penny is going
to drop, wouldn't it be
nice if we could simultaneously
put war into context?
Like how the hell did
some kid once strap on
a flame-throwing device,
point it at a bunch of
other kids just his age
and pull the trigger?
Then 10 years later
those people suddenly aren't
the enemy and we're
eating their exotic foods
for dinner.

Vietnamese?
Chinese?
Japanese, German,
Italian, Korean, Southern,
Mexican.

Enemies or cuisines?

What? We've got
to parachute into some
remote village and shoot up
the natives doing their
laundry down by the
river so we can discover
hot sauce? Do we require
any more evidence that
sushi to realize we've
been victims of parasitic
mind control?

Scientists have been

executed by Christians
and Christians ethnically
cleansed by Christians,
and on and on, and
what perpetuates these
things, yet we don't
know, and could even be
totally content <u>not</u> to
know, and in my book
this is not acceptable.

So get this straight
—there are pyramids
revealing themselves in
Antarctica as the
ice melts and obvious
signs of previous civilization
which just simply
overturns the
scientific, historical
and religious paradigms
and just along with
this whole "parasite
thing," stuff is
crashing down.

You thought this book was about parasites? This book isn't about parasites!

This is about the reality that for the past 100 years, physics has been paring down all humanity deemed was that _substance_, smaller and smaller, atoms to particles to vibrations until it was proven there's actually nothing here.

Just space, and barely that!

Then we dishonor
the existence of
everybody else by
suggesting "the whole
thing of <u>nothing</u>" is
becoming <u>overly populated</u>.
And there's a huge
pyramid in the middle
of Illinois that hasn't
even been excavated
because the evidence already
points to something
pretty weird, and there's
another in Bosnia, same
thing, hush, hush, and
all across the planet,
          hush, hush.

THAT's why I am writing this out by hand because nobody is going to believe what I write anyway.

Parasites dominate this planet 4:1.

# Really?



The United States would be the **melting pot** of peoples from around the planet SHARING parasitic <u>hitchhikers</u> brought <u>with</u> <u>them</u> safely in their guts.

Just like ANTs, infected with virtually microscopic liver fluke eggs, are driven by mind control to climb tall blades of grass and wait there to be consumed by a cow or a deer, this behavior is limited to high moisture zones, so the most horrifying species of parasites can't travel beyond their <u>ecosystem</u> of particular hosts living in close proximity.

Therefore, those stay put, and one must <u>enter</u> the ecosystem to become infected and a part of the life-cycle. However, some <u>CAN</u> travel because they bring their self-sustaining <u>eco-system</u> <u>WITH</u> them, such as small pox, AIDs, lice, fleas, bed bugs, viral this and viral that, bacterial this and fungal that. Some species are so stealth, they stir no symptoms.

Many, I contend,
are <u>so</u> stealth, they
are **yet** to be
discovered — I mean,
humanity does not know
they even exist.
It is entirely possible
that each person is
a cocktail of unknown
parasites like a totally
unique ecosystem
unto themselves.
Imagine flipping through
photos of every <u>insect</u>
<u>type</u> with a Dr. Seuss

variety of feet, hands,
wings, eyes, noses,
sensors, antennae,
abilities, talents, strategies,
colors, stripes, rainbows,
diets, synergies, symbiotics,
habits, living quarters.
Now imagine all the
ant types (thousands) and
spider types, reptiles,
birds, amphibians and
mammels. And fish!
And things with exoskeletons.
And eggs. Every
second: eggs and more eggs,
eggs upon eggs, green
eggs too.

Now bundle it all up
and stuff it into
Noah's ark. Then take
_four times_ the quantity
of all that because these
are _the parasites_, which
require a **host**, and surely
God created them too,
and barely any parasites
could survive free-floating
in a flood, while that
part was somehow **not**
brought up. So it's mostly
just **ludicrous** and
maybe even a **hoax**.

Meanwhile, science
is no better than
religion in terms of
explaining things.
Which came first,
the parasitic wasp
or the cockroach?
Which came first, the
pig tapeworm or the
pig? Darwin, who
charted minor variations
in species over time
based on survival of
the fittest, and postulated
that species _may_ beget
species, admitted that he
just invented the idea
without proof.

The fossil records do not bear this out. The monkey to human theory, Darwin would have been the first to reject, had he known it would be established as scientific fact. What the fossil record across 4+billion years shows instead is 4 main cataclysmic planetary events where approximately 90% of existing life forms went extinct.

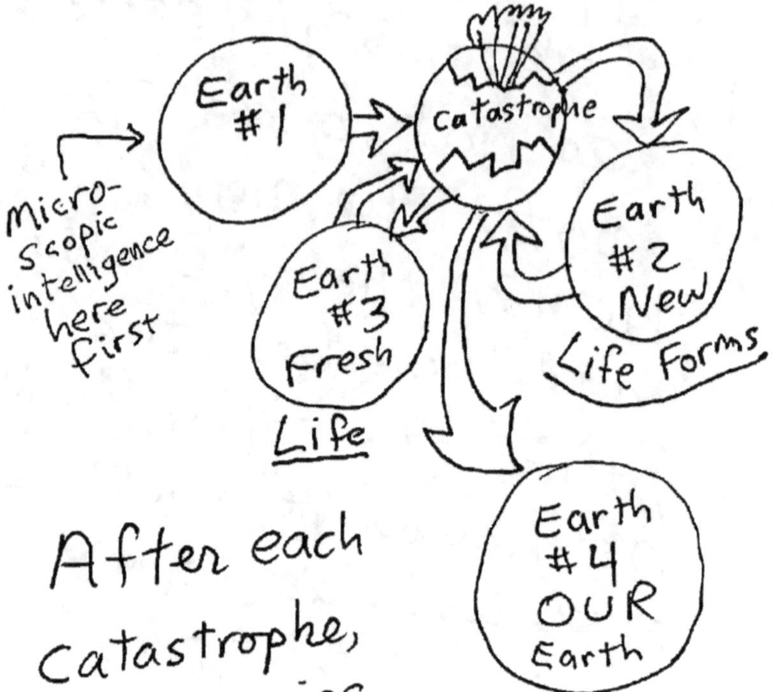

After each catastrophe, new species just "appear" as if dropped here from another planet. Humanity, same thing, appearing on the planet like a crop circle embossed across a British field over night.

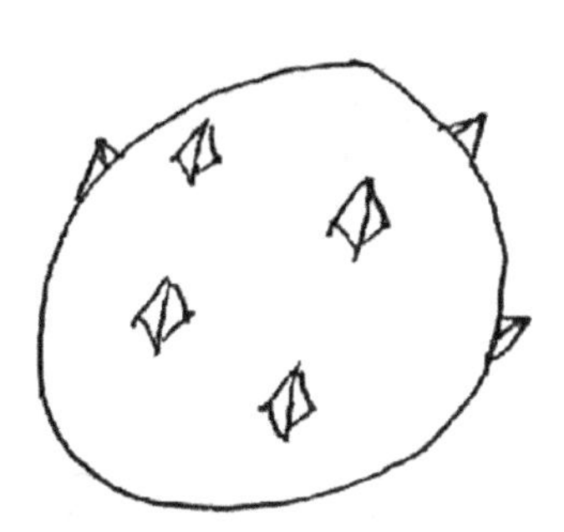

Plus, there are pyramid structures all across the Earth, not just 3 or dozens or hundreds, but __thousands__. Not only are they representative of mathematical equations, but astronomically positioned, not just individually positioned, but __placed__ in relation to planetary energy grids and not haphazard.

Not to mention the MANY megalithic stone monuments and walls and buildings, some now under the sea, some underground, some frozen in Antarctica. It's all coming to light, the bogus hoax of everything assumed to be grounded in Truth and fact, including the idea that Americans, mostly immigrants from everywhere, are minimally infested with parasites.

In case you are still
reading, the ^coming truth is
plainly visible:



• The <u>New</u> <u>Medicine</u> is
barely here. What's here
now is "irrelevant medicine"
which is being surplanted,
as what's relevant from
<u>old medicine</u> crashes into
<u>new Medicine</u> like
plate techtonics creating
wondrous mountains.

- Physics proving that <u>nothing</u> is the substance of what's here is overlapping medicine and the power of thought and emotion.
- Archaeology will soon finally tell us truthfully where we came from.
- The old things are falling away.
- The last thing for these bullet points is the amazing reality and existence of parasitic life.

"Definition" is what makes a parasite a parasite and turns a flower into a weed. Pull back slightly from the definition and all life is somewhat parasitic in nature.

The whole of reality is so chock full of LIFE, it's a continum of so much overlapping activity that it's like a boiling cauldron.

We are not going
to be able to
separate you
from it. As the
camera lens focusses,
enlarging what's smaller
and smaller, all the
tiny pixels you thought
were you is actually
mostly bacteria.
Reverse direction to
view what's larger and
it's like lifting up a
stone revealing a thousand
ants, yet within seconds
every single one vanishes.

They know. Even the most micro of micro particles run through a physics experiment demonstrate the awareness of being watched. These things must be factored — everything **You** know with everything **I** know. We've got to pool our resources. Start talking — **fast**. What do you know about planet Earth 2.5 billion years ago? Think, man, think!

How and when did these microscopic bacterial creatures get inside of us? I'm thinking it could reach back <u>that</u> far. Somebody brokered a deal. One side took bones and another side took meat, which they draped over the bones, then a third party took a cannon and shot primordial slime into it until the whole thing started to breathe. Right?

Is there a more fitting explanation? And then some of the slime dripped down man's leg and THAT divided into the parasitic wasp and a host cockroach, while the wasp took form first, and in that split millisecond, it devised a brilliant strategy to get the upper hand. And then the slime within man, and wife, likewise divided, forming into internal organs, right? Within →

the slime were micro-
scopic spores flown
in on meteors across
millions of years like
energetic plastic beads
of unreleased potential,
which gave birth to
worms so stealth
they could go on safely
reproducing in absolute
bliss in every season,
while man was forced
to earn his bread by
the sweat of his
brow.

Then the aliens came
down to visit and
saw that it was good.
They thus divided the
people by appearance
and set them into
giant holding pens we call
nations, and gave each
a scroll telling them
their origens, each
scroll varying widely
in explanation. What
could go wrong?

Then logic beget
logic beget logic and
with each begetting, the
whole thing moved further
from the truth.



Until one day,
little pieces begin
to collapse, then
whole ice shelves
start sliding into
the sea.

As the core logic unRAvels backwards into its original finest threads, people begin waking in their beds, jolting up in the darkness as if by electric shock and asking **WHY**? How did all these other people seemingly get in charge?

For as long as anybody
can remember, it's
been the Scrolls
guiding humankind
by their abiding light.
Then as if another
brighter light flicked on,
dimming previous
revelation, we see
now we've been
encapsulated in a
tomb. While the
upper eschalons from
the Illuminati on down
imagined
they'd been feasting, really,
they've been feasted
upon.

There is no new Divine ordinance triggering humanity's latest shift, no new economic, no new race, no new borders, no new anything. Just the same old ancient fact that primordial parasites rule the world because they weren't just here first and don't just own vast tracts of prime real estate; they _ARE_ the real estate.

Gently slide your fingers across your skin (yes it's a SKIN) and wake up with the realization that you are more **them** than you. From Day One they've been pumping their bodily fluids into yours to perfume every square micrometer from head to toe, and back, with their desires, not yours.

All those things that
you do, exactly as
you _don't_ want to do
it? It's as if you're
in a TRANCE, isn't it?
All those self-serving,
spiteful, jealous, critical
voices which just suddenly
pop into your thoughts?
Now it's suddenly
hilarious, ain't it?
You knew it all
along, that shit-talk
wasn't really _YOU_!

you knew you'd
see it for what
it was when the
phony imposters faking
humanity as the <u>NOT</u>-self
appeared across your
television screen
and more guns
might be purely irrelevant,
and irreverant, towards
advancing the more
wondrous cause.
    And the EXACT OPPOSITE
has been perpetuated as
THE TRUTH, and you

have anticipated the
day when the primordial
mud scales fell from
your eyes, because you've
scratched forever at them
without success and
by nature we can't
get it done by ourselves
because it requires a
kind and patient friend-
soul to gently take you
by the hand and do it
for you, so blind are
          we.

It's a riddle, as I said
before, and one not
put upon you to solve
yourself, same as
what you will eat today
appeared as if by magic
hands from elsewhere.
We are no longer
working from the problem
and then murdering others
to acheive the solution.
I myself have managed
to free myself ever
so slightly of my own
parasitic load, which

puts me ahead of it
by a fractal which
has allowed me to claw
my fingernails into a
crack in the veneer.
And if it hadn't
been _me_ pulling back
this curtain, it would
have been somebody
else, so blame _them_,
not me. Blame the
Pope, blame Hillary Clinton,
blame the Republican
Party, blame Mao Zedong,
just don't blame
me.

Because you <u>can</u> see it now, can't you? Blame Mike Pence, because you can see it now, his broken antennae on one side where his blood was sampled to confirm he walks about in a trance. Feel up there on your own head. It's broken isn't it, that one antennae? Oh for shame! For all the enemies we've killed without, only to find them living within.

<u>God bless</u> Mike Pence and now say three Holy Mary's. None of this is his fault or your fault and we can't fault Dr. Oz, not Dr. Phil either, not anybody.

Carry on, forget what I've said, everything is perfectly back to normal. There's no pyramids anywhere, nothing under the sea, or ice, or on Mars. Hey, the Beverly Hillbillies are on!

Look! It's Jed and Ellie Mae! OMG, Gilligan's Island is up next and today has got to be the day they will be rescued. I mean, pull up a chair, rest your feet a minute! I'm older than I was ten minutes ago and absolutely senile.
Back in my day, we knew how to get rid of intestinal parasites and I'll tell you how if you can sit back and rest a minute.

Now it's not all
that <u>irrelevant</u> to
ask yourself –
"Which came first,
the <u>human</u> <u>soul</u> or
the leaders of the
        Taliban?"

which came first,
the poppy flower
fields or the U.S.
    opioid crisis?

"which came first, recent
human civilization or the
awareness that the
planet Earth rotates
        the sun?"

"Which came first,
everything you know,
or everything you
don't know?"



<u>And who's smarter
about it all?</u>

Gilligan or The Skipper?
Mary Ann or The Professor?
Thurston Howell III or
Mrs. Thurston Howell III?
Galileo or the Catholic bureaucracy?
Team A or Team B?
You or IT?

<u>THAT's</u> all I'm saying! We might want to start <u>pooling</u> our resources. What do <u>you</u> <u>know</u> and how can you help?

Ah — Jethro is back, and Granny too, and she's hoppin' mad! Granny's about to give something a good whoopin' and if we know anything for sure, Granny'll give it a good whooping.

# Chapter

# 5

# Para·norml

So—
About one year ago,
a new client named Angela
started coming to see
me for colonics. She was
already well-versed in
colon hygiene and familiar
with what goes on inside
the body. For several months
she received one colonic
per week. In the late
fall of 2016, the evidence
presented itself that her
body was host to a
tapeworm. Somewhat busy,
by early January she was
eager and ready to get
into it.

Angela was not like any other client I had ever worked with. For one, she was intuitive and astute regarding the various layers enveloping the discovery and removal of a tapeworm.

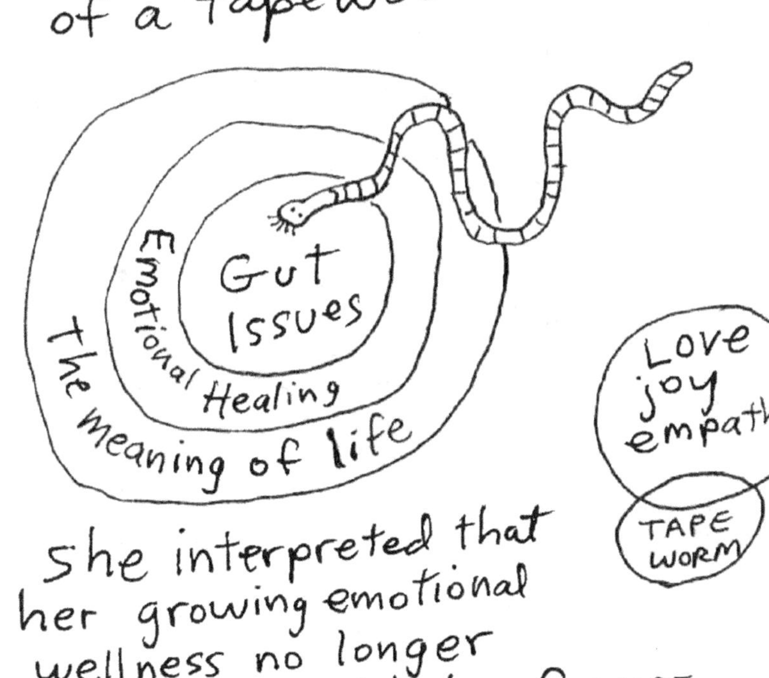


she interpreted that her growing emotional wellness no longer resonated with her former self.

Some part of Angela had awakened and this part of her told _me_ what _she_ was going to _do._ What she didn't know, was that I had just envisioned for _myself_ a similar thing – a 30 second snapshot of me with less itching, dryness of eyes or puffiness.    She _mobilized_ as I _watched_:

One week passed.
No tapeworm came out.
Two weeks.
Three weeks.
Four.



Angela received about 15 colonics across the first month and every second we watched for a tapeworm to make its exit. What neither of us anticipated were her day to day mood swings and up and down energy level shifts.

The client and the therapist can both view what's coming out during the colonic. One day, Angela said:



"That's a worm!"

I made an attempt to clarify: "No, that was a large glob of mucus. The colon will secrete <u>mucus</u>, like the sinuses, as a <u>self-protection</u> to coat and/or remove harmful gunk, poisons, and invaders."

Mucus is normally not seen by people because it gets FOLDED into what appears like ordinary poop.

MUCUS → inside

A colonic breaks it APART

I explained that a tapeworm would utilize mucus as DEFENSE protection against beneficial bacteria. Bacterial waste is hydrogen peroxide which can kill worms. A tapeworm secretes ammonia to keep bacteria away and mucus can form a barrier between the two.

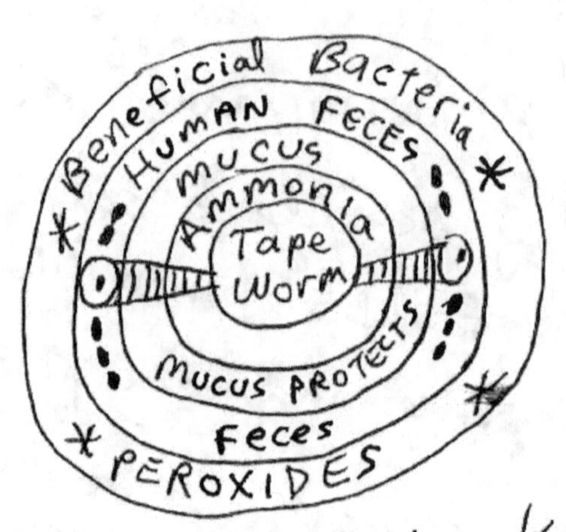



The tapeworm thus keeps access to the human's feces, while avoiding peroxides. The worm requires no stomach because its food is pre-digested. Mucus in the colonic water was a good sign because the tapeworm might be weakening. Plus, Angela's mood swings could be from more AMMONIA from the dying worm absorbing more into her blood.

Angela begged to differ. She thought she had killed another kind of worm

and THAT was wrapped in mucus.

I said: "Angela, the odds of you hosting two types of worms is just not very likely."



The next day, Angela said: "There's a FLUKE!"

I thought that it looked like a red potato skin, but Angela hadn't eaten red potatoes. After her colonic, Angela pulled up photos of liver flukes on her phone. Sure enough, she was right. I asked her, "Angela, WHERE did _you_ pick up a <u>LIVER FLUKE</u>??" She suggested it was because she was from Mississippi, which initially sounded far fetched to me.

she suggested that the old plantations had long been a kind of breeding ground for the giant African liver fluke. We Googled that too on her phone and the number of such cases in the U.S. was about **zero**. So we just sat with it, the possibilty that Angela might have a tapeworm, a giant African liver fluke **AND** another kind of worm which at least one had died and we saw it enfolded into MUCUS.

I started telling my other clients what was going on. One of my clients researched it and bought a ten pound bag of DIATOMACEOUS EARTH, which is a powdery silica. The edges of the particles are sharp as razor blades and glass shards. My client gave me 8 lbs., and I gave it away free to my clients in little bags. Pretty soon every client was releasing bizarre shapes and textures and I was snapping photos with my phone camera.

Then Angela released
a seven inch long, dark
brown glob, folded over
on itself like made from
rubber.

Giant African liver
fluke? At first we
said nothing. We just stared
at each other. "THAT,"
I said, "was an OCTOPUS!"
By now, I was taking the
diatomaceous earth and
nothing unusual was coming
out from **ME**! What I
mean is, we tend to think
others could have worms,
not **US.**

And so it was that something ELSE strange came out in Angela's colonic water: pea-sized pods with translucent coatings.

I asked her, "WHAT have you been eating?"
She said, "Nothing like that!"
I video taped it and snapped pictures: 200, 300, maybe 500 passed. I stomped my feet. Tears of shock & sorrow flew from my eyes. These were fluke EGGS.

Later, another client released those _exact_ _same_ kind of eggs. She was in her early 30s. Long before she had come to see me, she had experienced sudden skin rashes and headaches along with terrible constipation. About 100 eggs released during her colonic. I was telling another client about this, a fitness instructor. She said, "Well I hope *I* don't have worms." Just then, a white jelly blob with black dangling legs came out.

← Actual size

The photos which I
am about to show you
were taken in my office.
The demographics of
my clients are all across
the board in terms of
age, race, affluence
and level of health.
These photos were taken
from a random sample
of five clients' colonics.
I can't photograph my
colonics, but I too have
been releasing all the same
worms. I would conservatively
estimate

that these past 3 months
I've been releasing ten
worms per day — yes,
about 900 total. This
experiment is not over.
I call it an experiment
because no matter WHO
you are, addressing parasites
within the human body will
always be an experiment.
Other colon hygienists from
across America also report
that they see worms
coming out from their
clients.
            Angela is the Prime
                      Mover

with all of this, truly
leading the way. She
has been at it for eight
months now and what a
priviledge it's been to
have a front row seat
for me to watch her
discipline, strategies and
persistence. I review some
of that later.
From the hundreds
of parasite photos, I've saved
140. For this book, I am
publishing about 50.
For every photo I took,
I missed many, because
either the worm came out
too fast or else
unexpectedly.

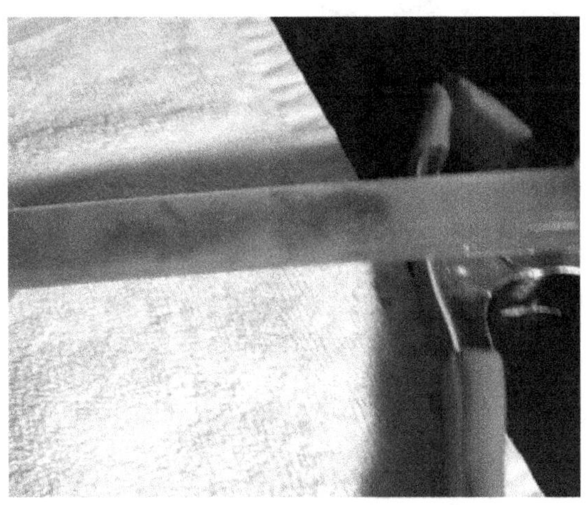

Note little appendages and how this floats as gelatinous,
not fecal.

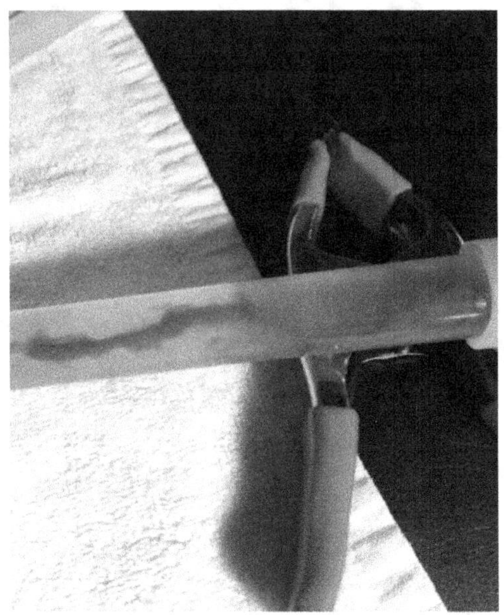

Obviously this jumps out and says: Worm! Foot long!
Popcorn! Cotton candy!

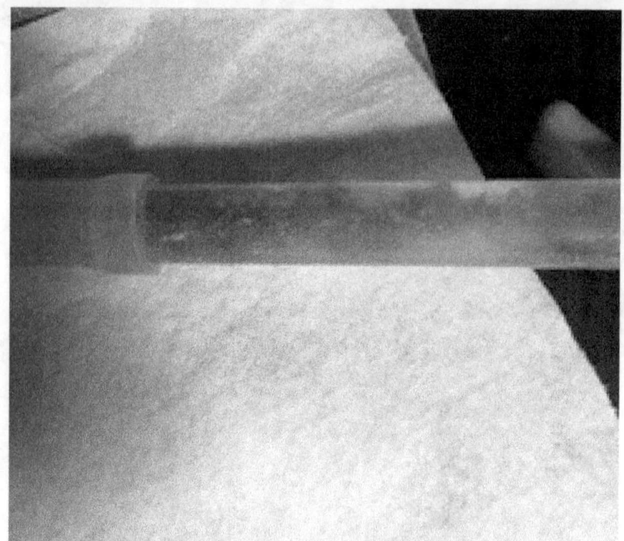

Previously I identified this as mucus, but there is most likely a worm behind why this all holds together. Like a caterpillar spins a cocoon, this monstrosity is productive with its time, spinning slime to make its bed.

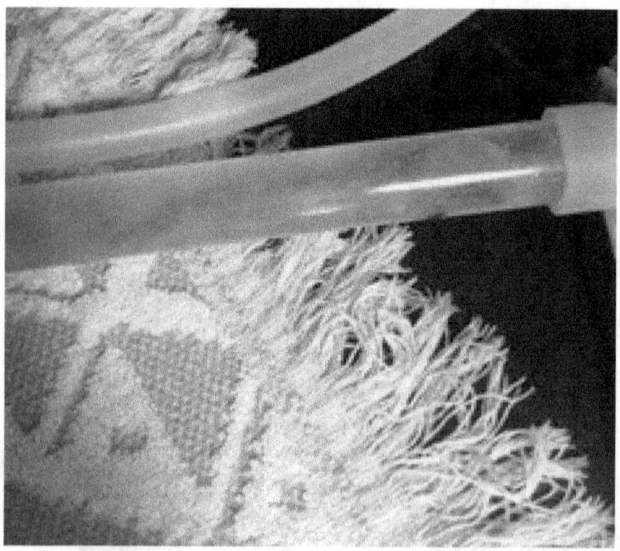

Same thing here, except this is a totally different TYPE of worm from the above, about 15 inches long. These two worms came out different days, same person.

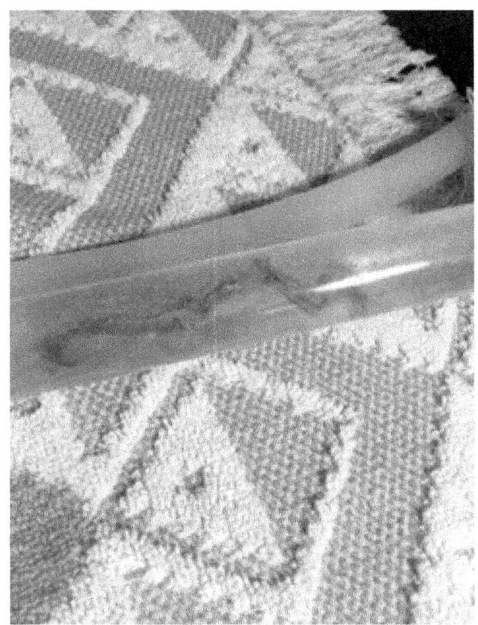

This worm is encased in a layer of mucus, about 9 inches long. We can see its handiwork stripping off like a layer of dead skin.

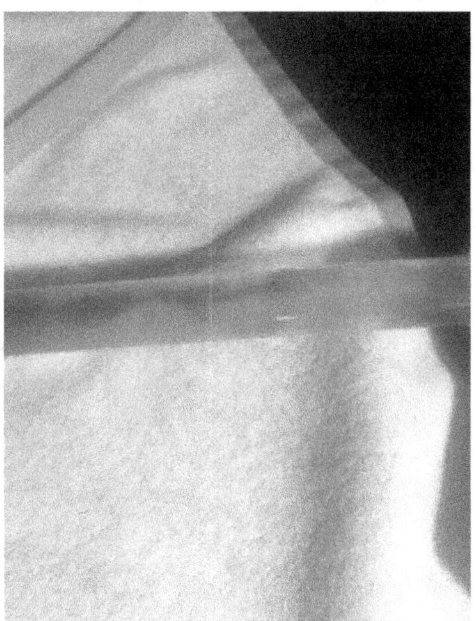

Note appendages and prehistoric appearance. These things also give off energy as they leave, which my clients feel at the same time I do.

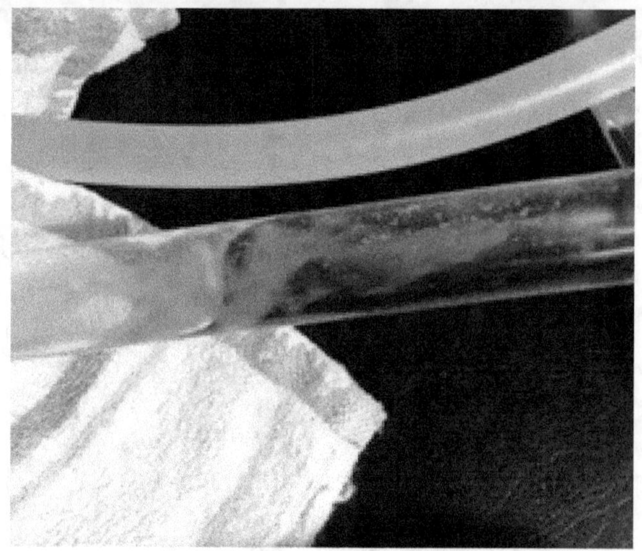

This is pure and simple, a worm, like a cobra, again, cloaked in mucus.

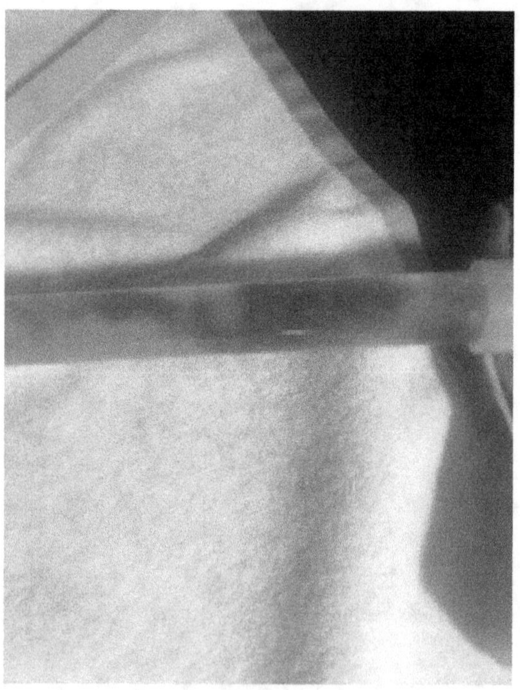

I would guess this to be in the FLUKE family, large frontal body, long trailing tail of some sort, unless it's coming out backwards.

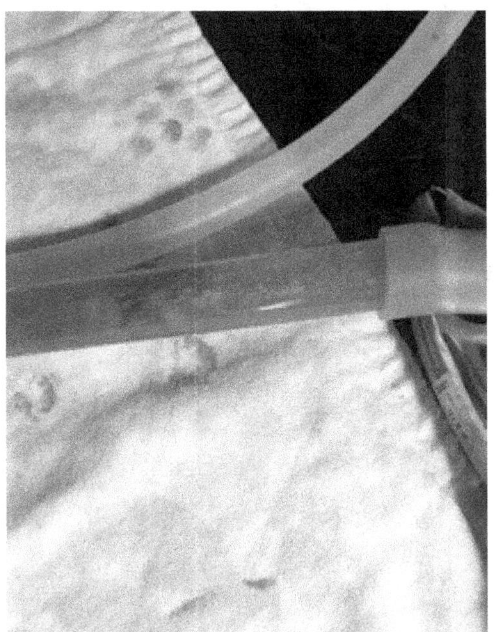

A lot of times, these things exit within a gush of brown water and you can't distinguish exactly WHAT it is, worms or poop. This one has two little air pockets clinging to it, with off-white mucus appendages.

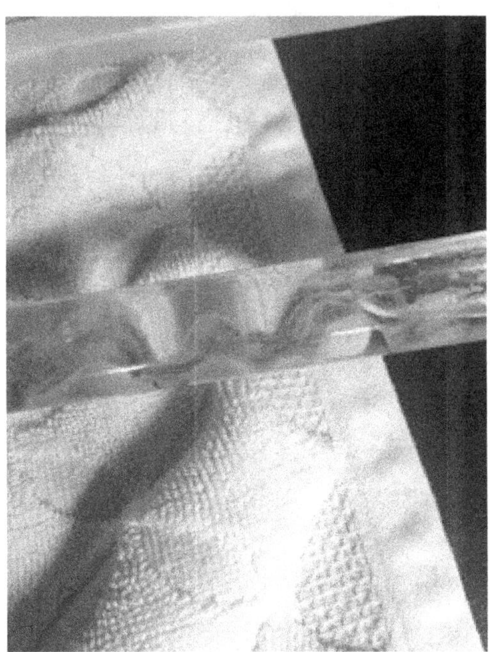

This isn't just one worm, but two, two worms in one!

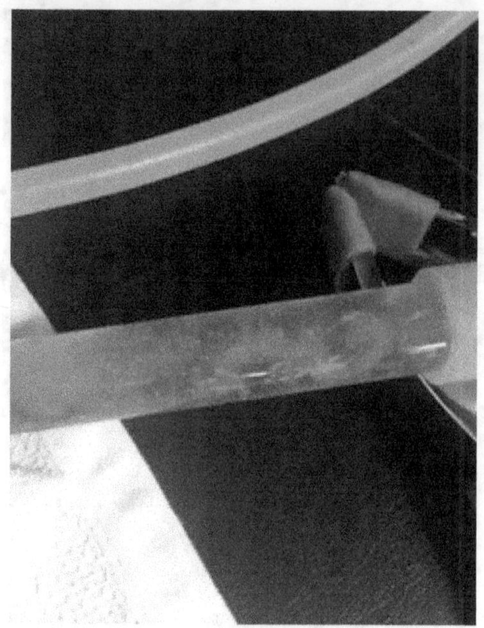

If this person wasn't on a parasite cleanse, we could say,
"Well, that's just a shrimp being chased by a minnow."

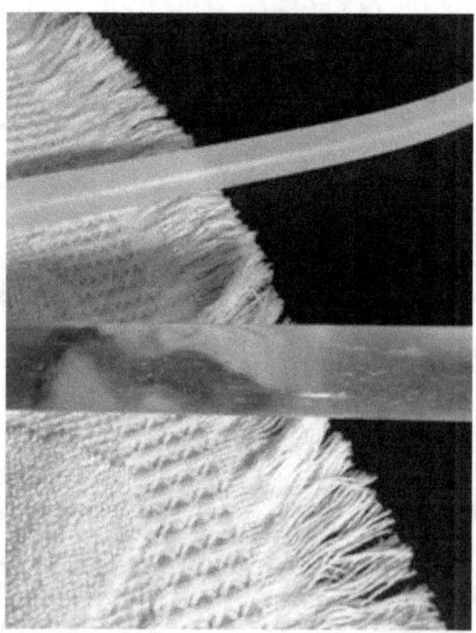

I saw this big boy coming through and said, "Say cheese!"

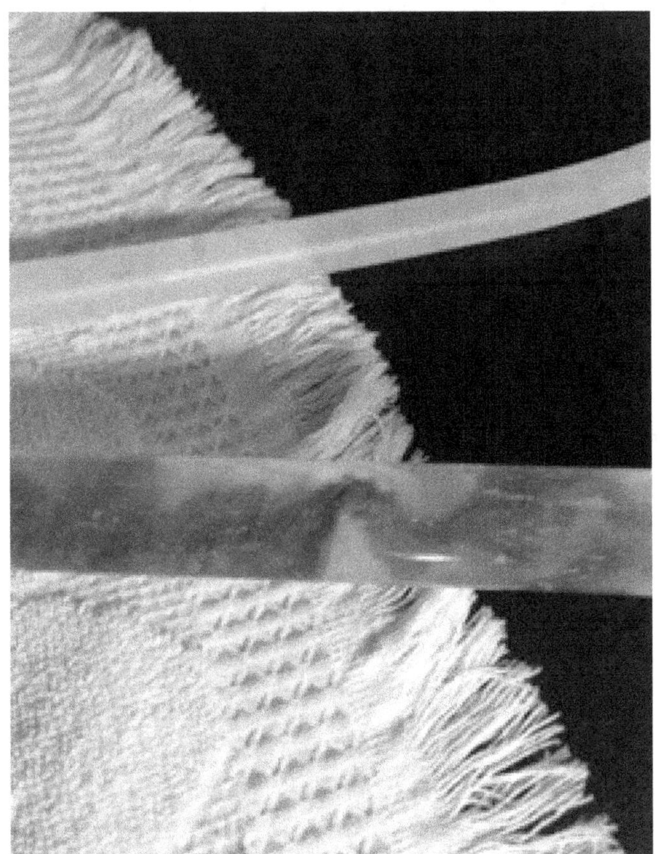

CHEESE! We can see the worm exposed smack in the middle like black tape. What's odd is that it has stuffed fecal matter into a kind of stocking. For a midnight snack, the icebox is pulled up right next to its bed.

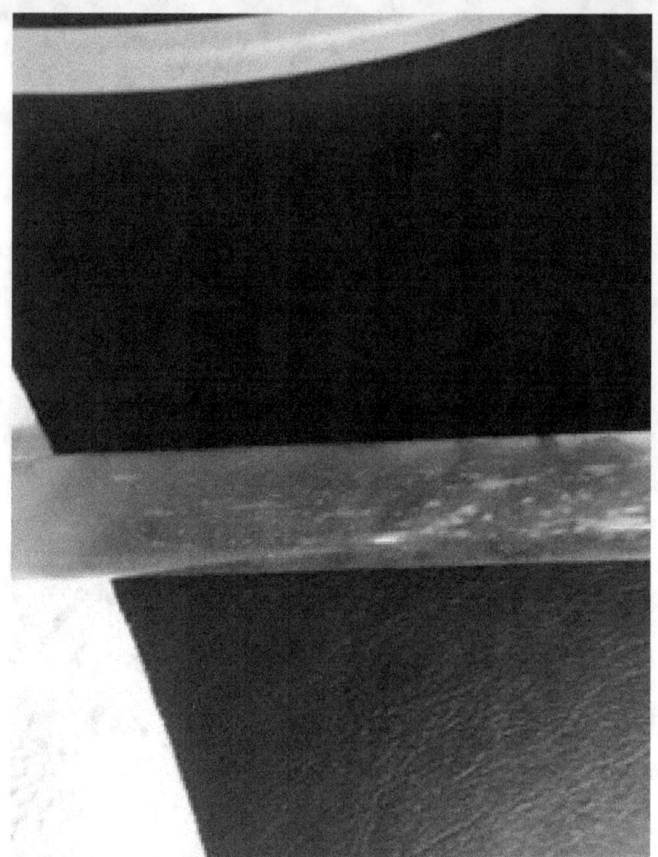

This fellow's been dead a while and trailing an orange cloud of slime. Keep in mind, what you have seen so far is what could exit in a SINGLE colonic. Next colonic, same person, then again, similar creepy stuff dressed for Halloween. Noteworthy is how the person removing this feels afterwards. Relief. The objective is to kill whatever it is and then to pull it out as cleanly and as effectively as is humanly possible. Right? That's what I would think anyway.

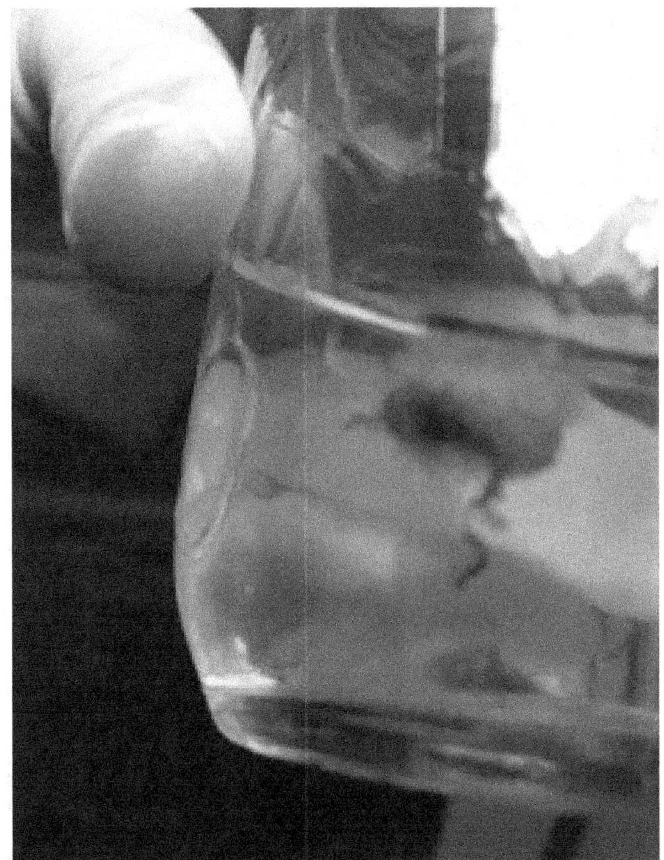

This lovely specimen was discovered floating in the toilet following a colonic. We Googled it. It's some sort of a fluke pod. It has mucus that's peeling off at the top and some sort of arm or leg or siphon appendage hanging out. We also observed about a dozen more coming out during the colonic, but this one we captured.

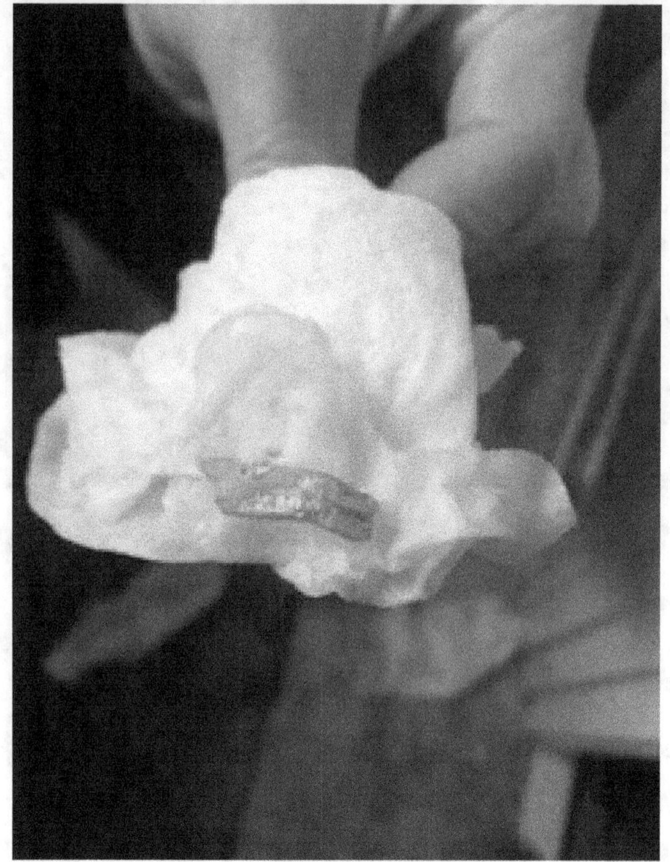

After another colonic, about 20 of these "shell things" came out into the toilet. My client Googled it because they all were identical and did not appear like any food recently consumed. She identified it as a blood fluke. To me, it looks like a cicada.

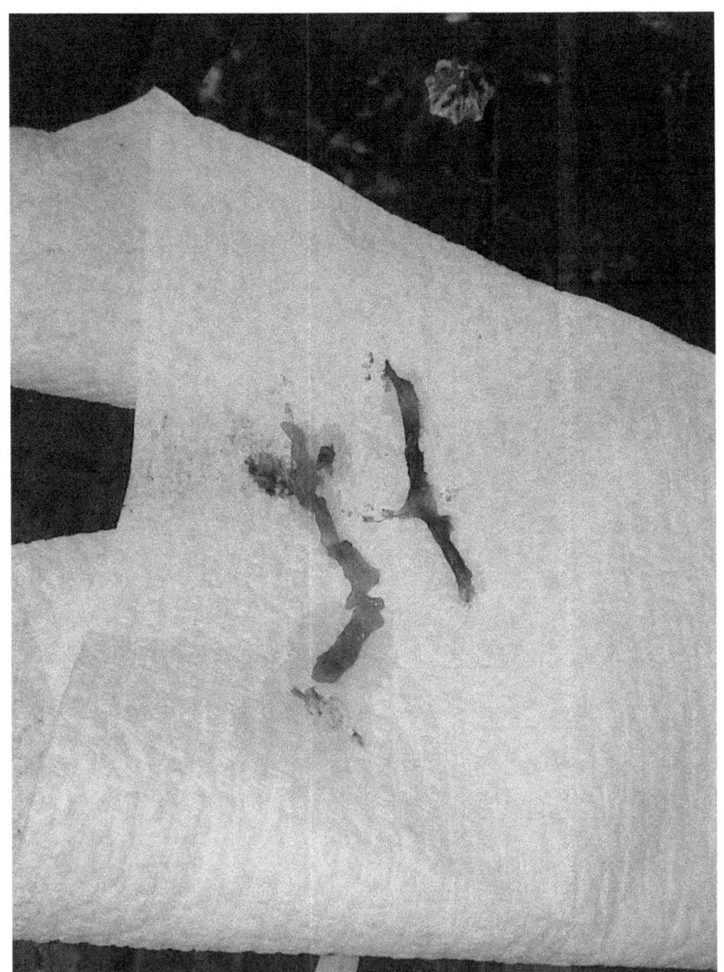

A married couple came for a colonic while on a parasite cleanse. The husband released no parasites during his colonic, which was his first colonic ever. He was relieved and guessed he did not have any parasites, then purged these into the toilet later, which he fished out and draped across a paper towel.

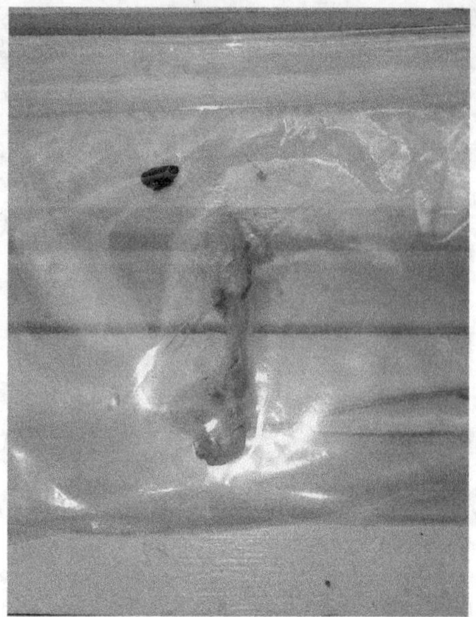

His wife also released a very similar worm later at home.
She put hers into a plastic bag.

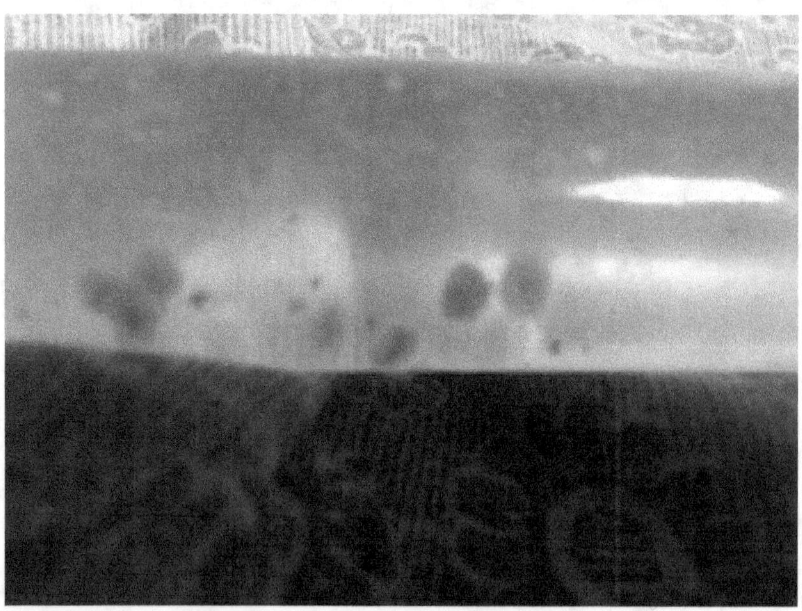

These are the eggs I mentioned earlier. You can see the dark
centers with a gelatin shell. Here we have seven eggs. Sometimes
the tubing would show fifty or a hundred pouring out at once. I
have film footage of it too, which I'll post on my website.

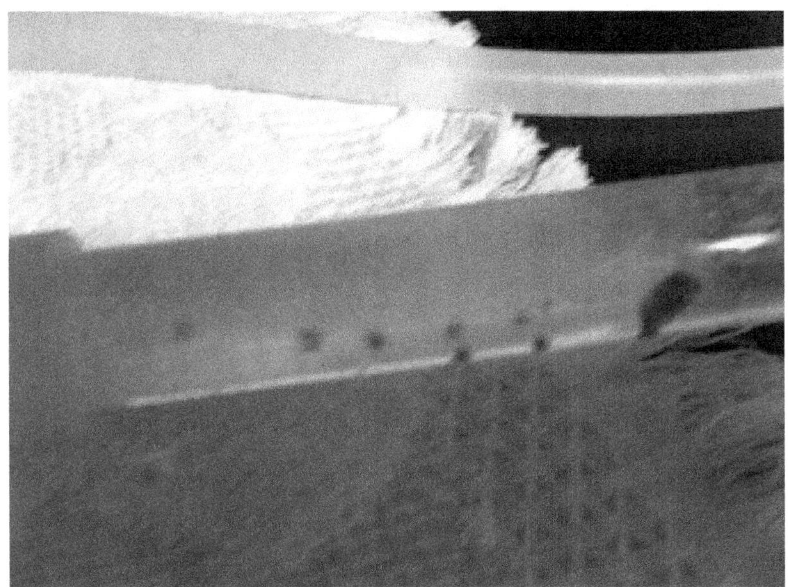

There go more! Eggs with a little fluke in tube at far right.

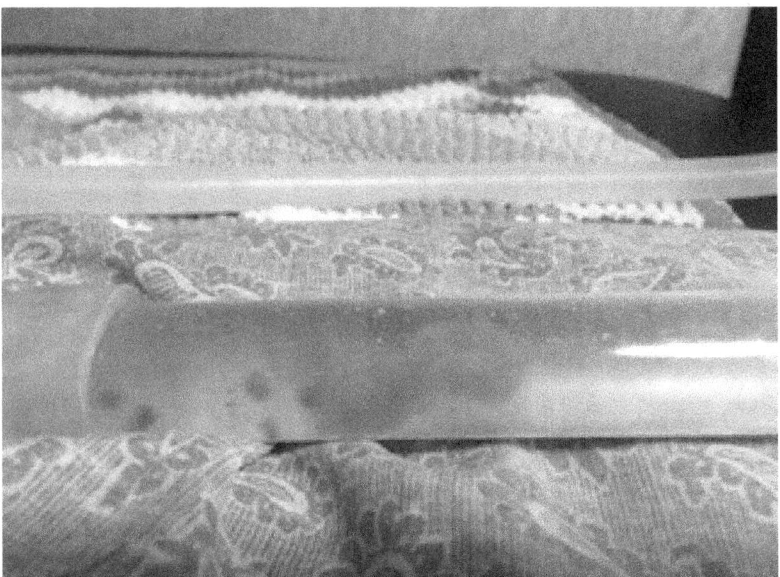

More eggs with another fluke at center. These eggs released from two different clients on the exact same day. Was it the phase of the moon? Was it dumb luck or just a random sample of two Americans, while similar eggs were also inside how many more people sitting at home watching television or checking their Facebook?

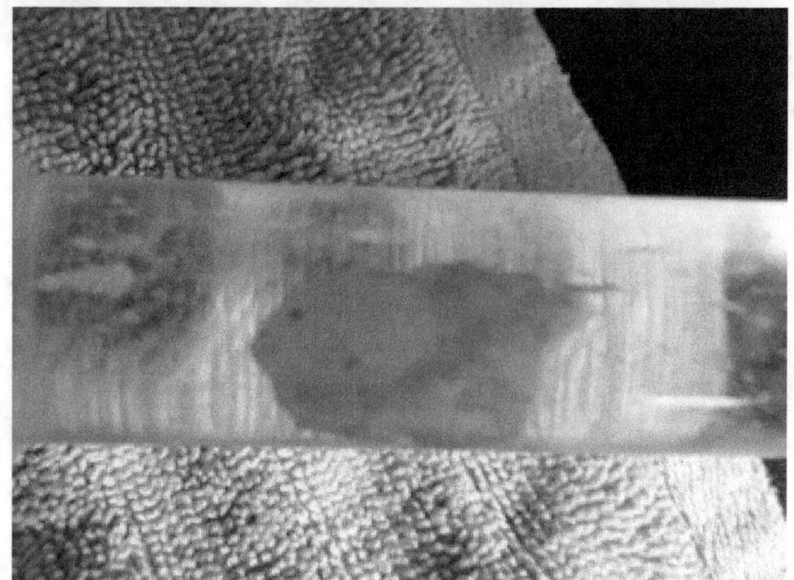

This is the very fluke which I identified as "a red potato skin." When we searched for pictures of flukes on the Internet, we were able to identify this as an adolescent stage fluke, for sure, pointy nose and all. The color is salmon pink.

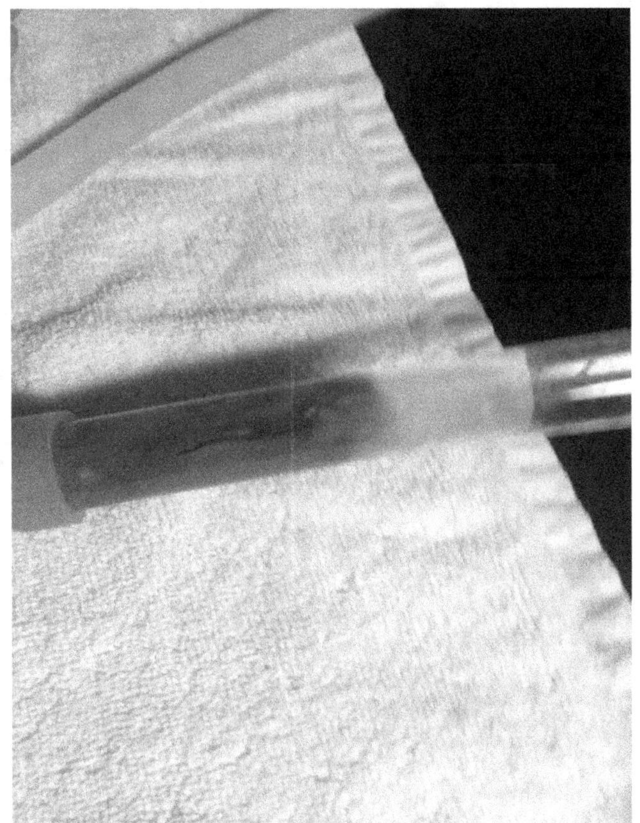

This is a very large adult fluke. I know it appears like poop, but it ain't. We have pictures of eggs, baby flukes, and adolescents, so there's no reason to wonder if there might be full grown ones too, maybe years old. Do they stay in one spot or move around? Why can't we feel them? Angela and I figured we saw seven of these come out in one day within 30 minutes of each other. They are flat when alive. Just yesterday, we saw ten more come out.

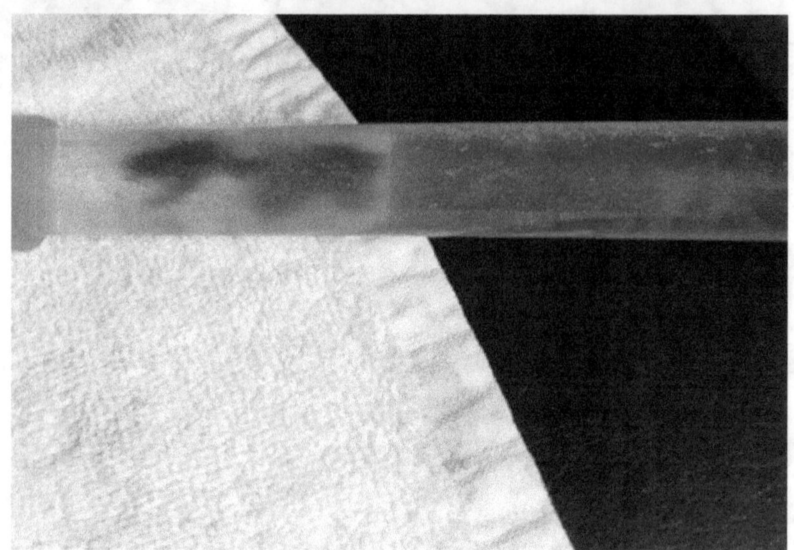

This was another fluke, but smaller so it wasn't folded into
the tube. What does it look like? T-Rex!

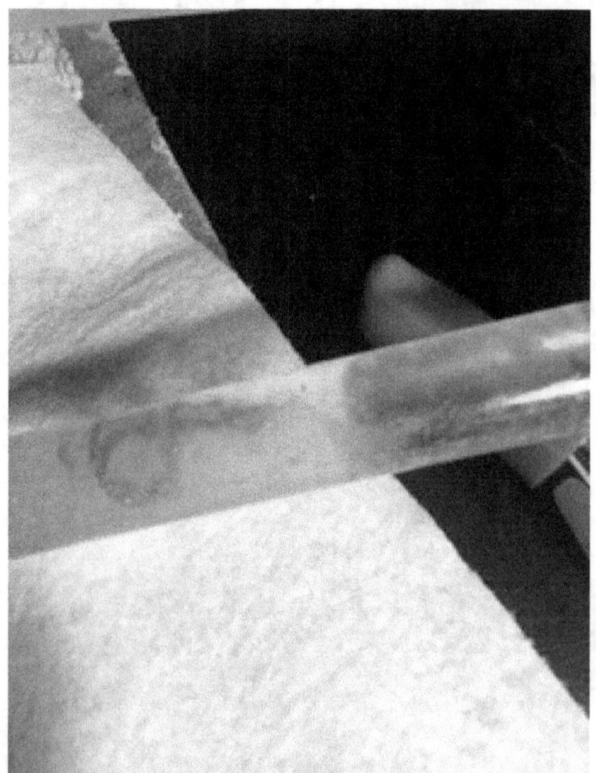

Can't tell if this is one worm or two in a double helix.

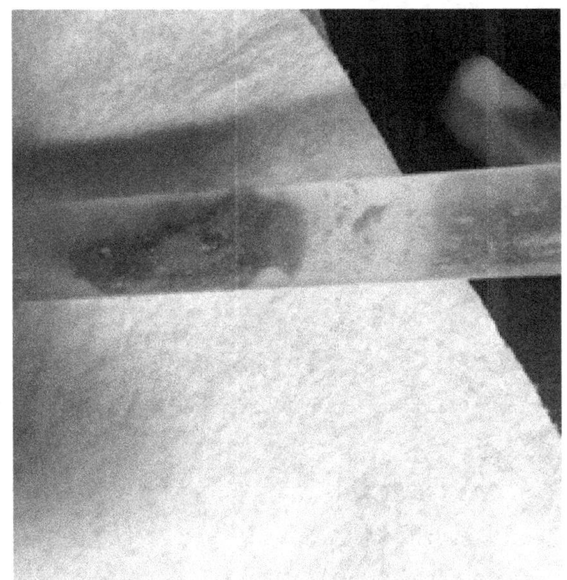

I love this guy. Looks just like a dead bird. Ca-caw!

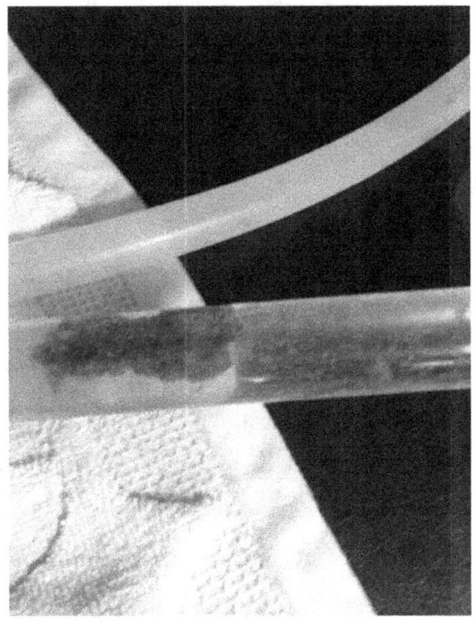

This one looks like the body of a crawfish. It's got little round balls on the underside. What did it look like when it was alive? You tell me! Here it is just a carcass. This might be only a section of one and the other half or two-thirds of it is still stuck inside the colon.

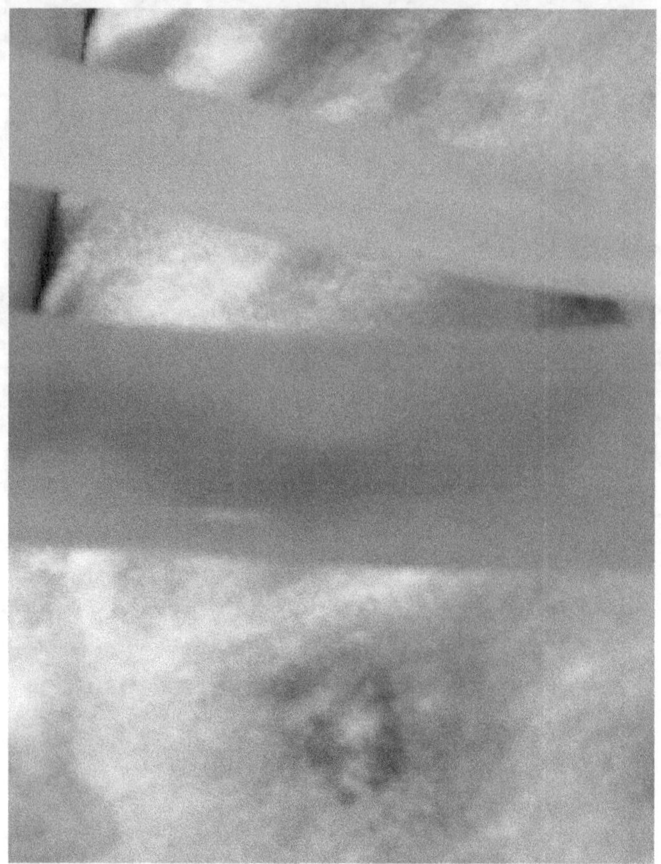

This one was hanging at the top of the tubing. It refused to drop out, so we couldn't see it in the clear view tube. It appeared like it was swimming, long as a snake (15 inches), when I realized it WAS swimming, not wanting to come out. I took video of it that I will post. Then it gave up and flew down the tubing like a rocket. A week later, this happened AGAIN. The second, identical worm stopped right in the view tube and then swam against the current like a wild salmon. I tried to photograph it, but I was so shaken I dropped my phone. Then it too vanished out and down into the sewer, thank God.

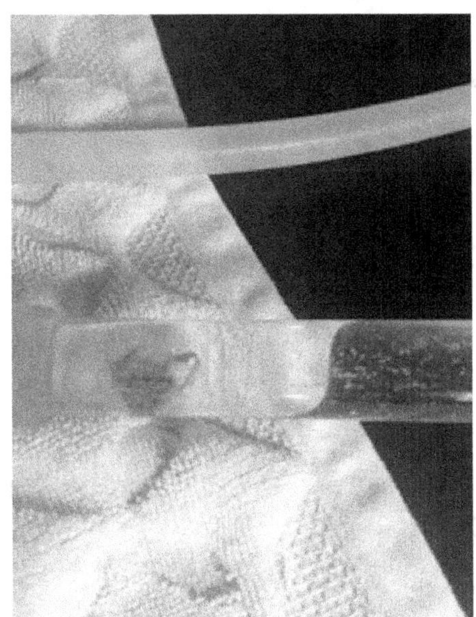

I love this guy. He is either all body with two arms or some kind of pod with worms coming out.

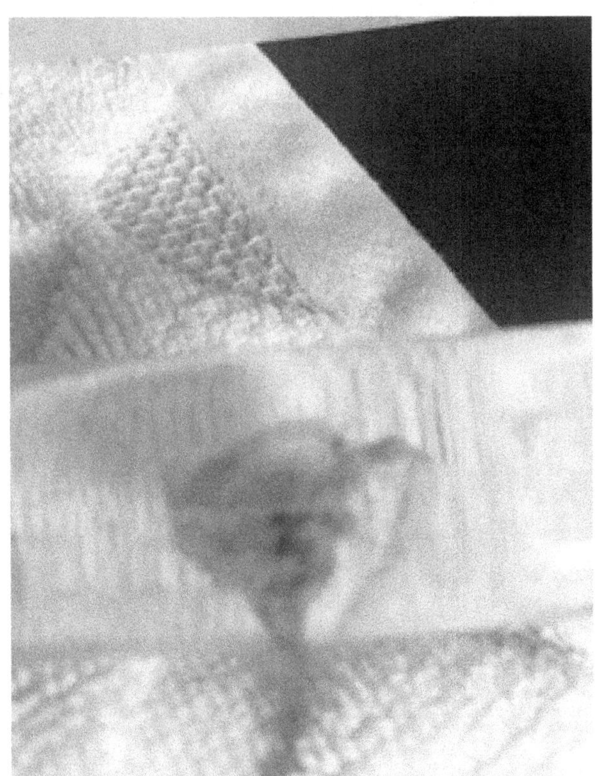

Here is another closer picture of it. I call him Lucifer.

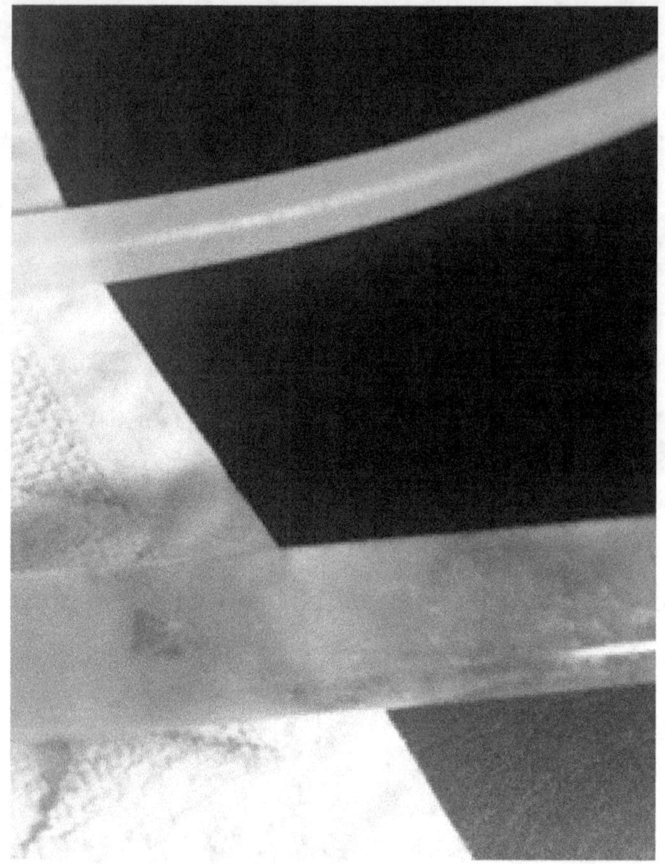

This is a very long decayed worm, but also with a young,
bright pink fluke.

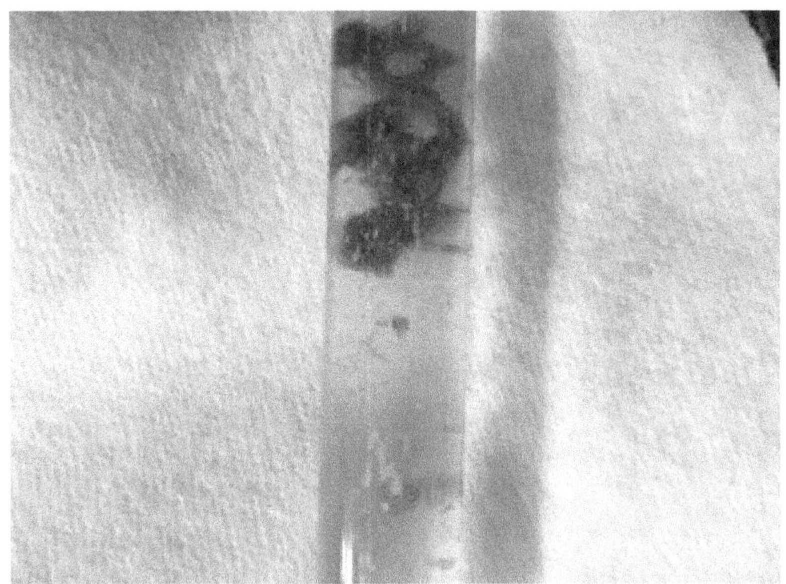

For some reason, these worms get into a tangle. Could be lying around all day and mating. On a bed of food. Also, have you noticed the wide variety? Most of these photos are taken of what's come out from ONE person. So you start to wonder: Are these things in ME? It's not like I casually said I'd do "a parasite cleanse." I myself decided to do an EXPERIMENT, see if these things were in me too. Not everybody is lucky enough to be able to do four or five colonics per week, to watch what's dying inside and floating out when you do certain things to kill worms. I have been unable to photograph what's been coming out of me, but yeah, same stuff. I'd estimate that I will see a Variety Show of 30 worms come out from me per colonic. I've seen about five, two-inch leech-like worms come out that looked identical to leeches I'd get on me as a kid swimming in lakes. How much smarter to live UNDER the skin. I'd estimate I've removed over 900 substantial worms in three months from me alone. Sometimes I will take a teaspoon of small-batch turpentine, not the commercial stuff, and an hour or so later I will FEEL worms moving in my legs, chest, and even around my eyes. Otherwise, I have never felt anything crawling under my skin. It feels like a bug is on my leg, but when I look, nothing is there that I can see. The crawly thing is UNDER the skin.

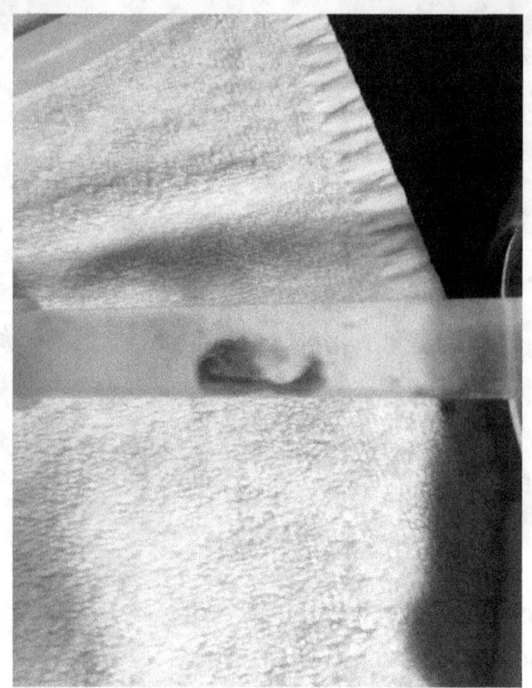

What's the etymology of that? A head, neck, bulb?

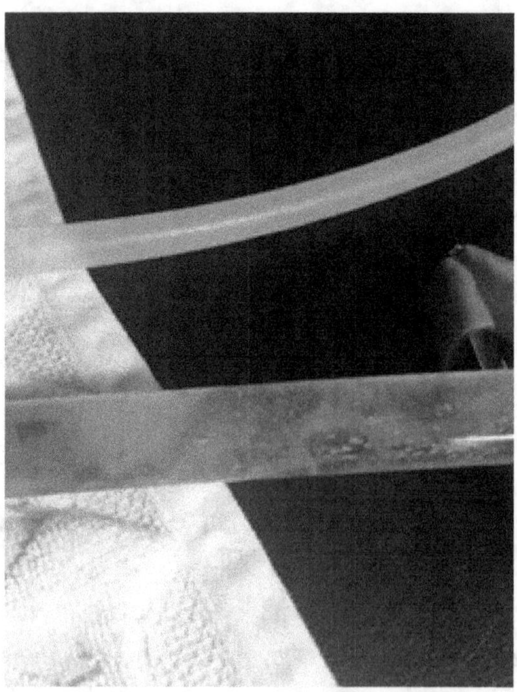

Another picture of a worm with little fluke trailing, both
life-cycles rudely interrupted.

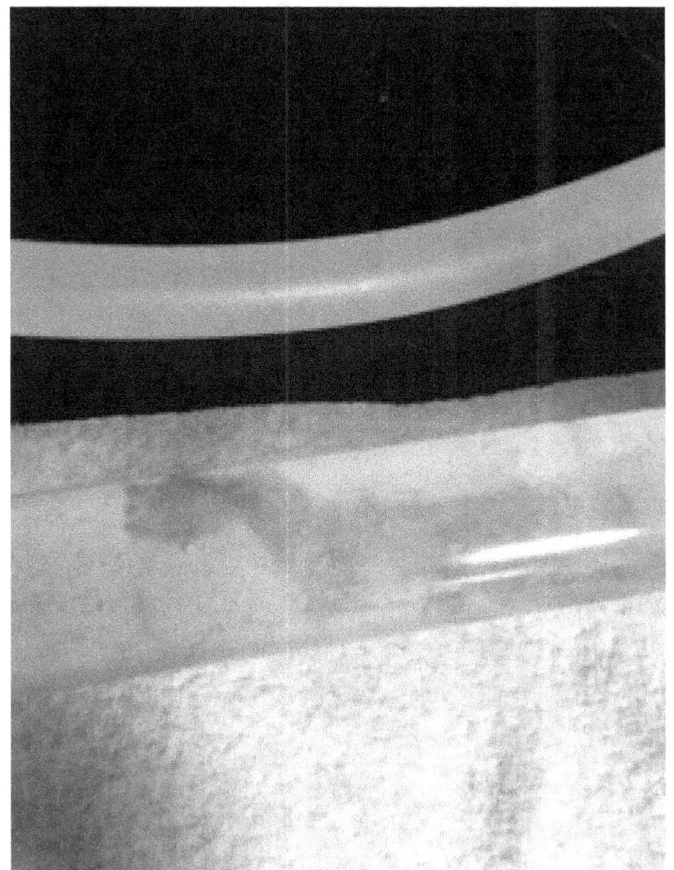

This appears like a head with a one-inch wide ribbon body, deteriorating into slime. This can get into the digestive tract, at or near the top, and the system will digest the worm because it's made of protein. This worm could have been hanging out ANYWHERE in the human body, died, was purged into the intestines, then digested like anything else passing through and now a shadow of its former self.

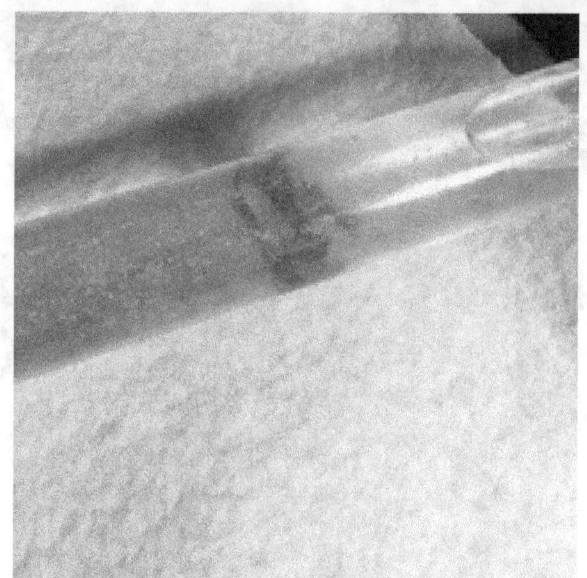

Same thing here. If you swallowed a dragonfly whole, it might come out looking like this, like a giant dead crumpled insect.

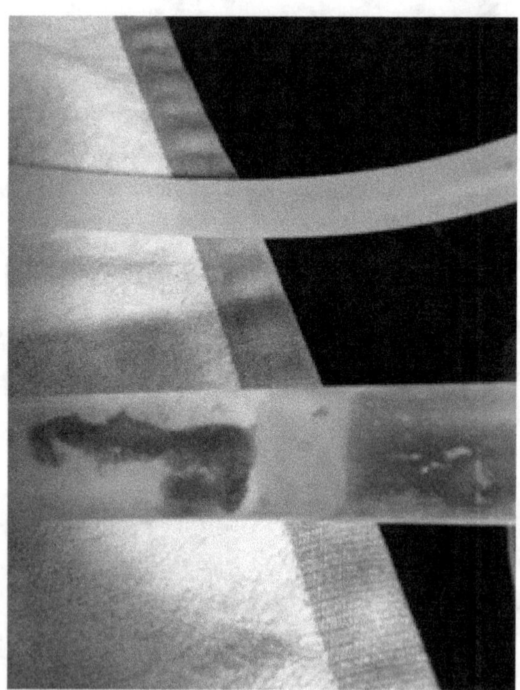

Seen enough? I have! This thing is half shrimp, half fish, half sea monkey.

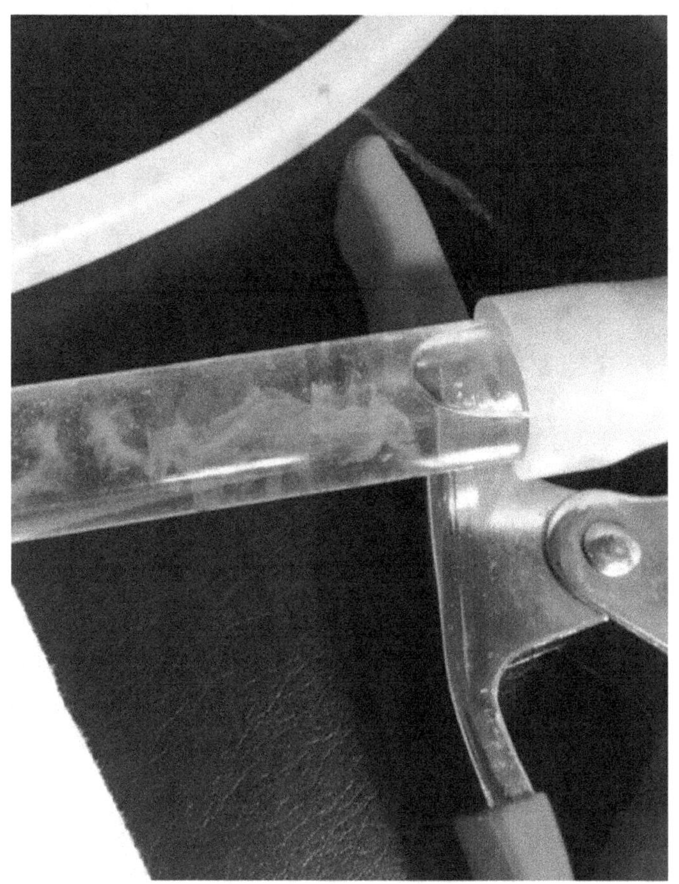

Some of these look like they have faces and legs. I see a goat. With a much smaller sea monkey. Two sea monkeys!

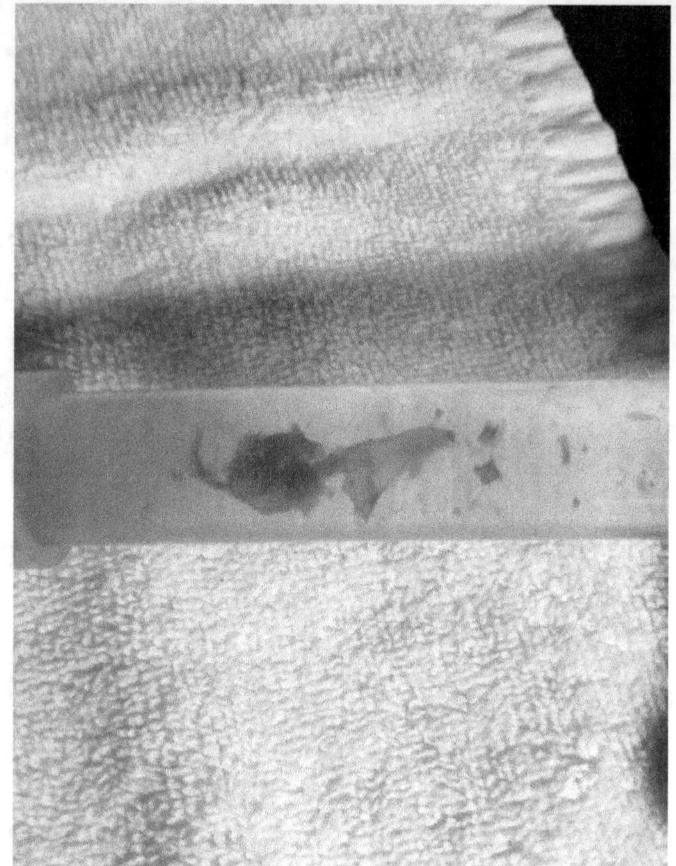

There's a baby kangaroo jumping out from a pouch that has an umbilical cord. If these creatures are asymptomatic, this kind of thing may not as of yet been discovered by science. And what are those two alien pods doing in front of it?

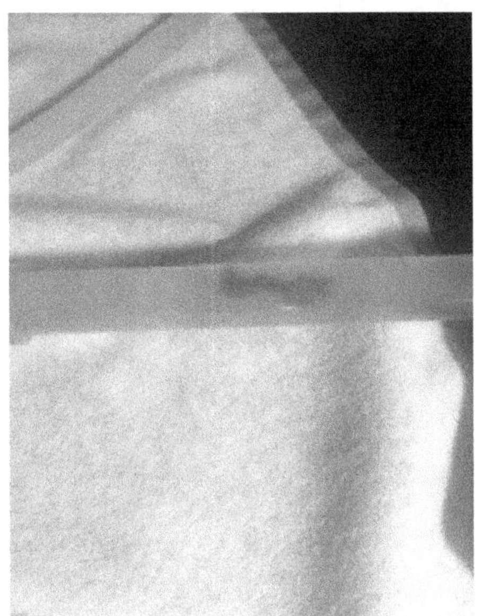

Just your run of the mill worm, nothing special, probably dropped dead in the pancreas or sinus cavity. Wherever it was, it's not there now.

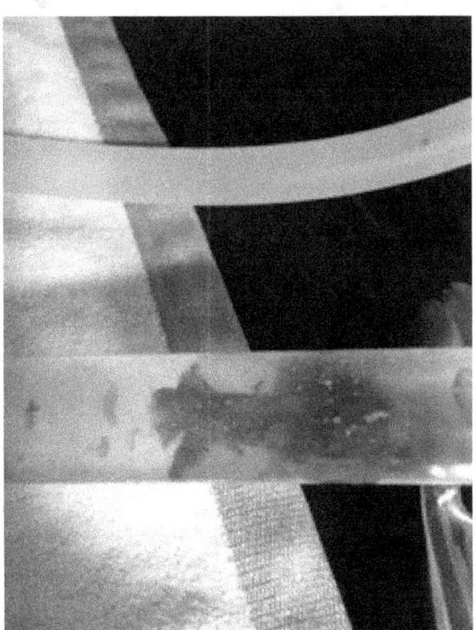

Another crawdad, bird, totem pole thing. It was once a baby, but big and juicy just a day or so earlier, probably thinking its own wormy thoughts.

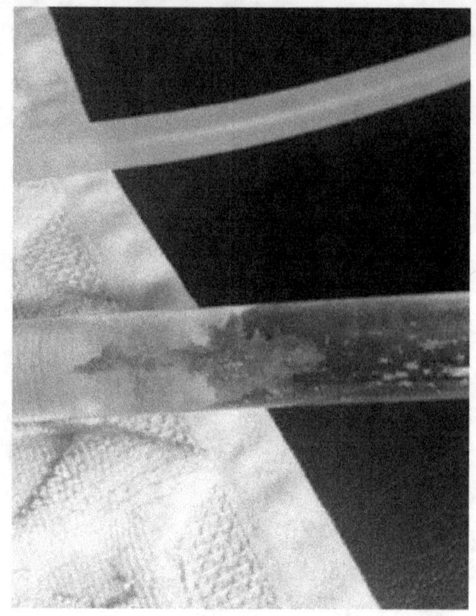

Flying fish reptililian?

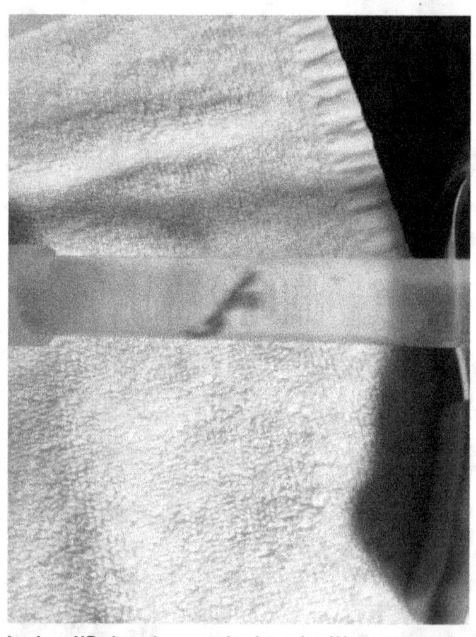

Boy running with ball? It doesn't look like much, but it's nothing you'd want in your soup. Clients ask me, "Where are people contracting these things?" From you! You imagine those wiggly shapes aren't in YOU? Everywhere you go, you are spreading little spores on door knobs, menus, at the pool, at the hotel, on the airplane. Passing them on to your dog. Where else you been lately?

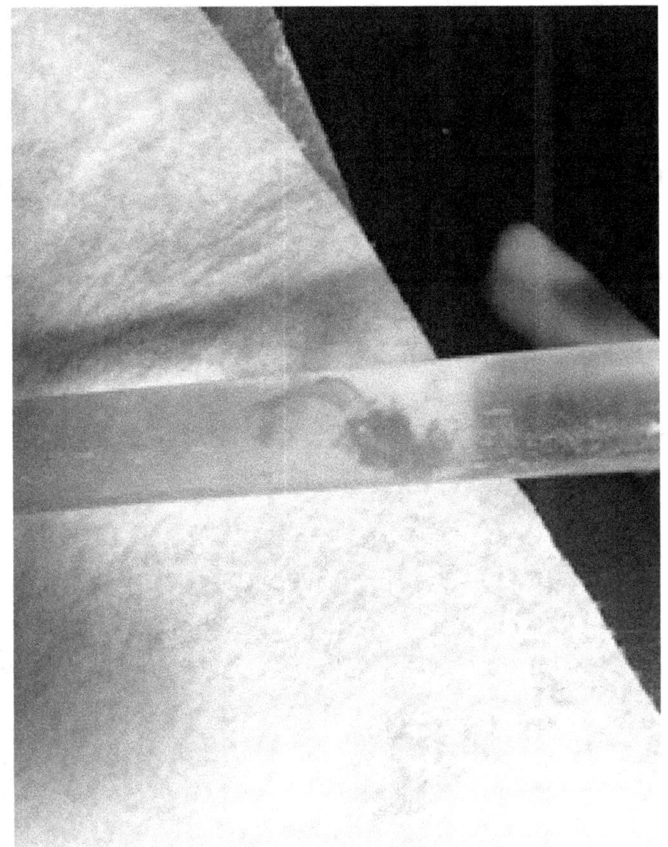

To me, this looks like one of those fish you find deep under the sea where there's no light. What's odd is that the shapes are often prehistoric-looking, reptilian insect-like. What's scary is that they also appear to be perfectly suited to our internal environment. If they come in every size and shape like from a Dr. Seuss book, they are likewise passing each other in the night. Our bodies are their ecosystem. Remember, parasites have parasites. Leopard frogs, which I used to catch as a kid, have multiple parasites and in this case, as far as these colonics are revealing, WE are the swamp.

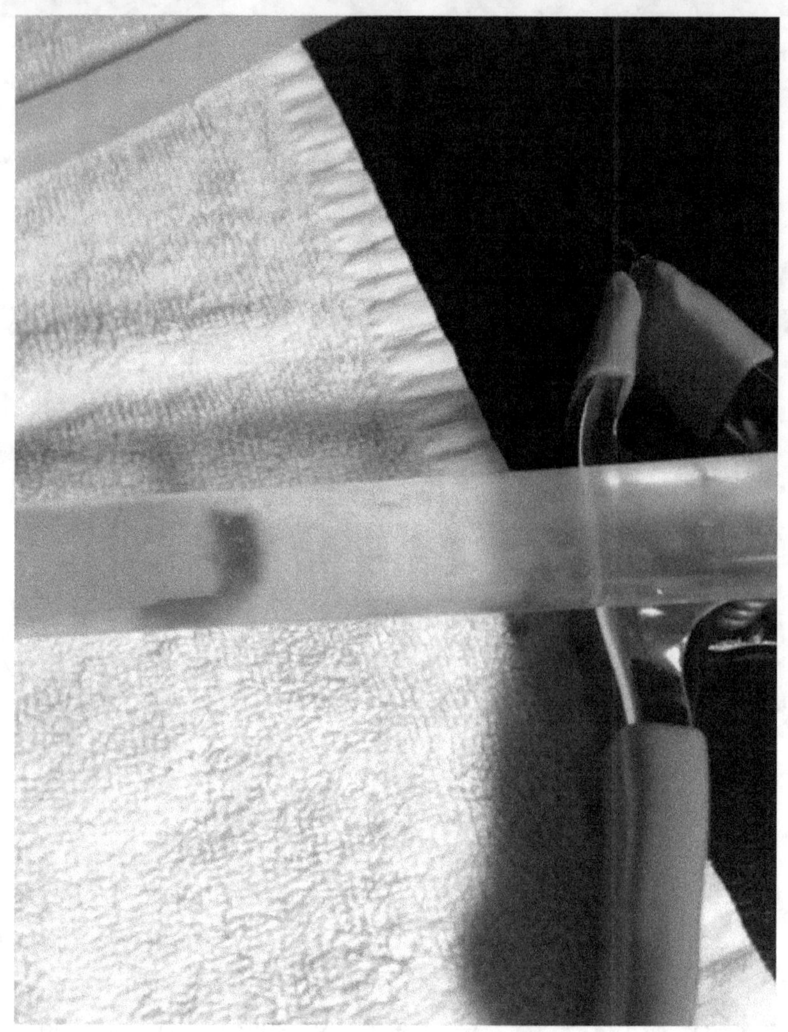

A more humble little critter. Aw!

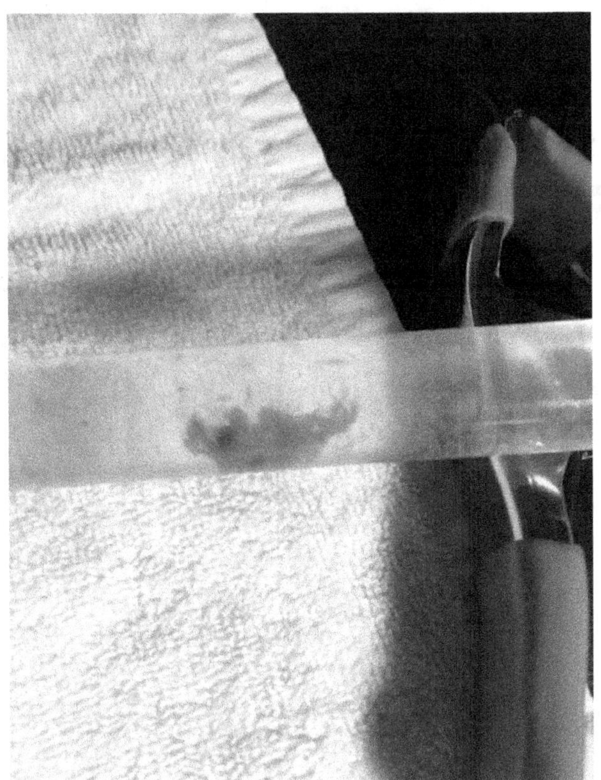

Again, the number of photos you've looked at so far can represent what comes out during a SINGLE colonic. I watched a YouTube video in which a parasite removal expert advised NOT to do high enemas or colonics during a parasite cleanse because that would "remove valuable minerals." That's laughable. These dying things are ROTTEN. And they stink. I can poop five times in one morning, do a colonic, and watch 25 additional dead worms come out. Dead worms in the bowel will make a person feel nauseous. If a person does a 7 day parasite cleanse, they ain't even scratching the surface. A three month parasite cleanse is only going to reboot THE PARASITES. Go slowly. Use water up the butt. Three months is better than nothing. Six months is the start of something. A year of doing some small thing every day to kill and flush parasites is the game. Nobody will do it if they feel nauseous for an entire year. Add water. Up the butt. At the very least, an enema. Daily. If not daily, every other day. Nausea indicates more water needed. Up the butt. Sorry, I didn't make up the rules.

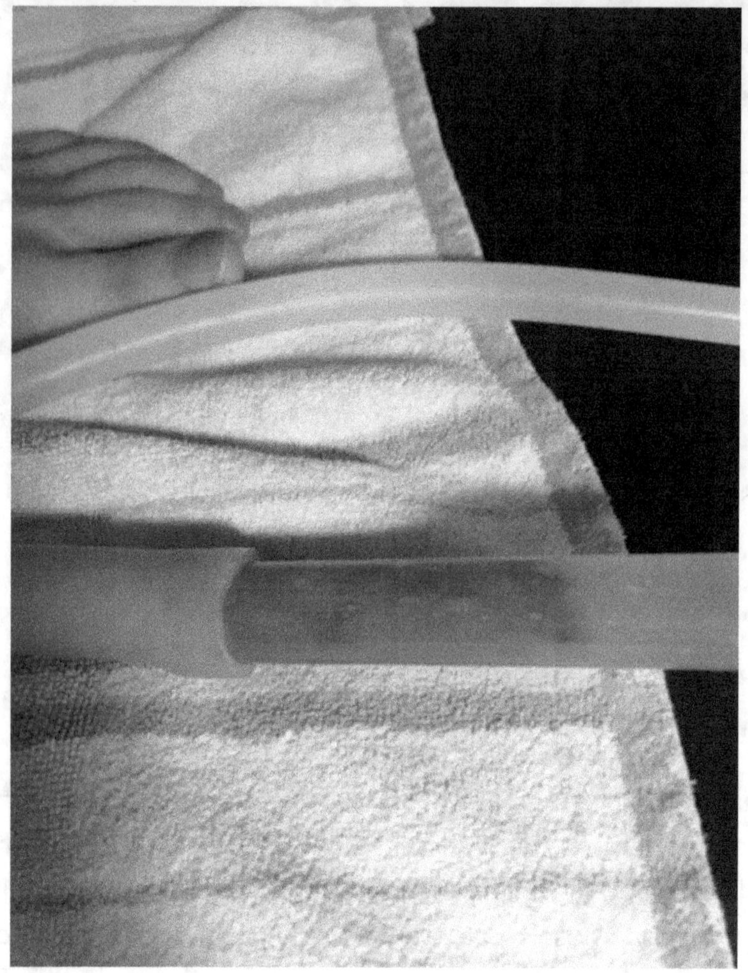

Gargantuan something akin to a railway train. If you haven't attempted a serious parasite cleanse, and then done twenty colonics, and think you have a better opinion about what this is, you don't.

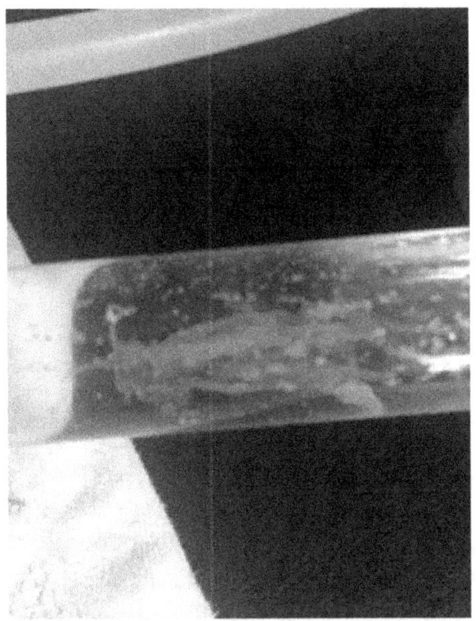

Grasshopper alert!

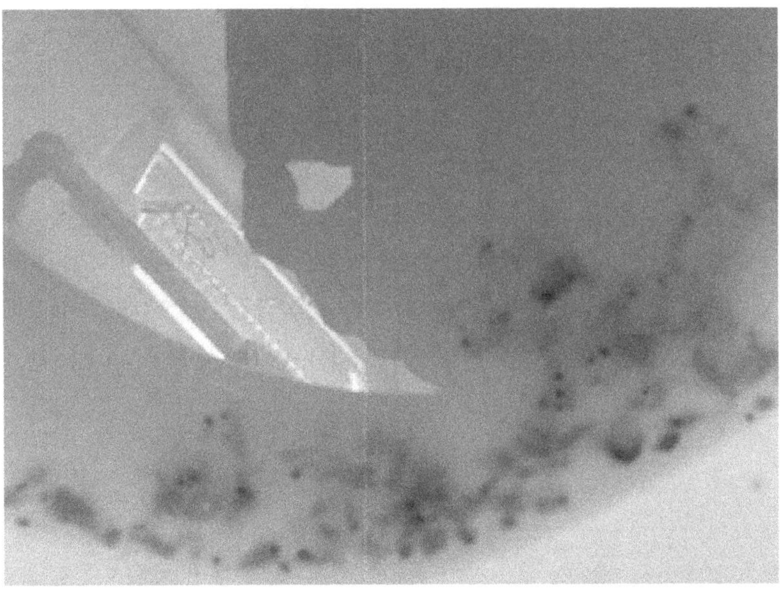

My client flushed and came out with this photo of what was in the toilet after her colonic. Little skeeter larvae with black heads. I said, "Well, that's something new and different!"

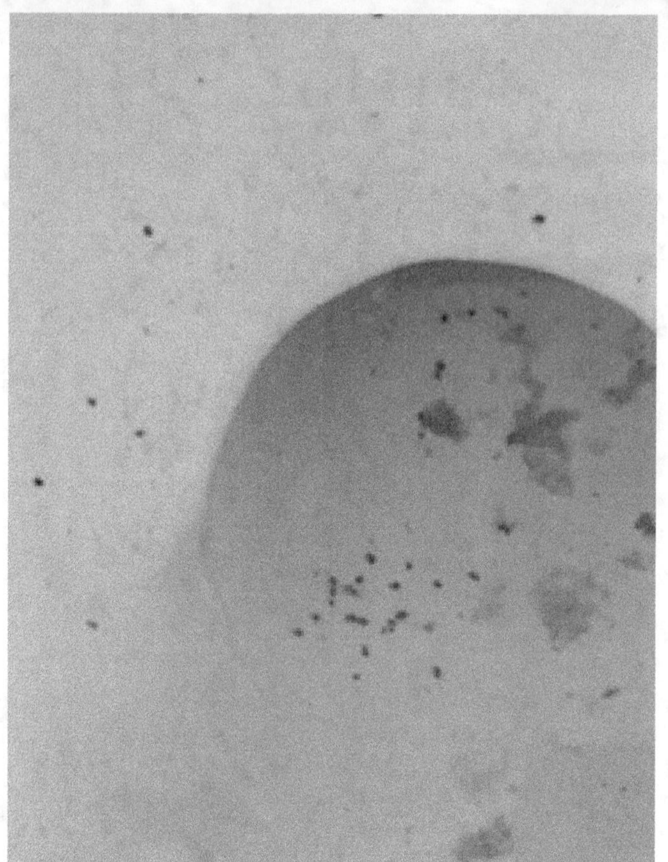

This is what came out in the toilet after MY colonic. Little black eggs that looked like flax seeds. I DO eat flax seeds, but these weren't that. Eggs. Never mind the wormy mucus also that came out, a mere fraction of my total "output" that day.

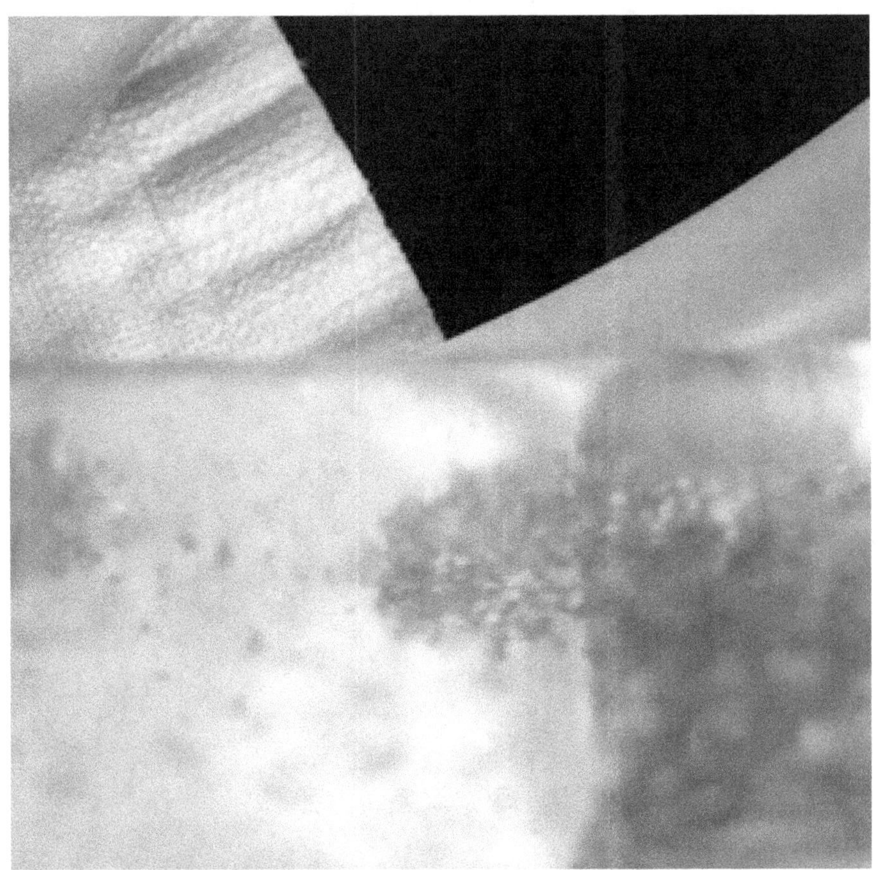

I have seen this, for years, coming out from clients. It appears like SAND that collects in the colonic tubing. Those are eggs. I'll confess to you the truth: I ignored it. I didn't believe it could be from larger worms. I simply remained in denial. Now when I see it, I say, "Hey, um, maybe you might consider taking diatomaceous earth every day for the next year." "How come?" they ask. "Well," I reply, "Just in case you have a few intestinal parasites, diatomaceous earth destroys the eggs."

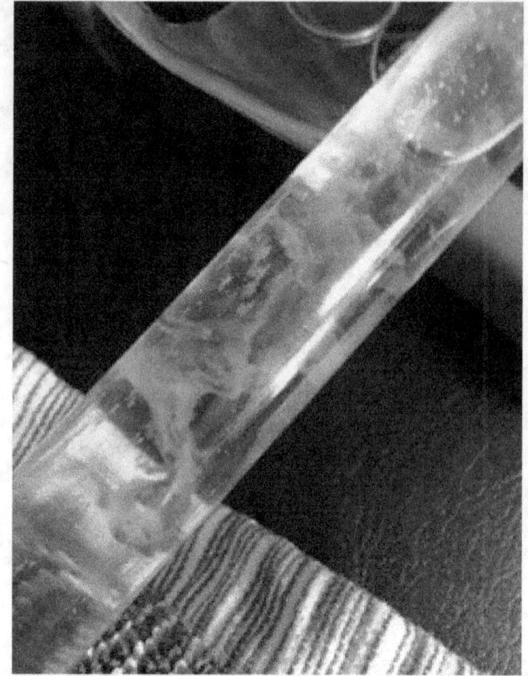

Huh! Creepy.

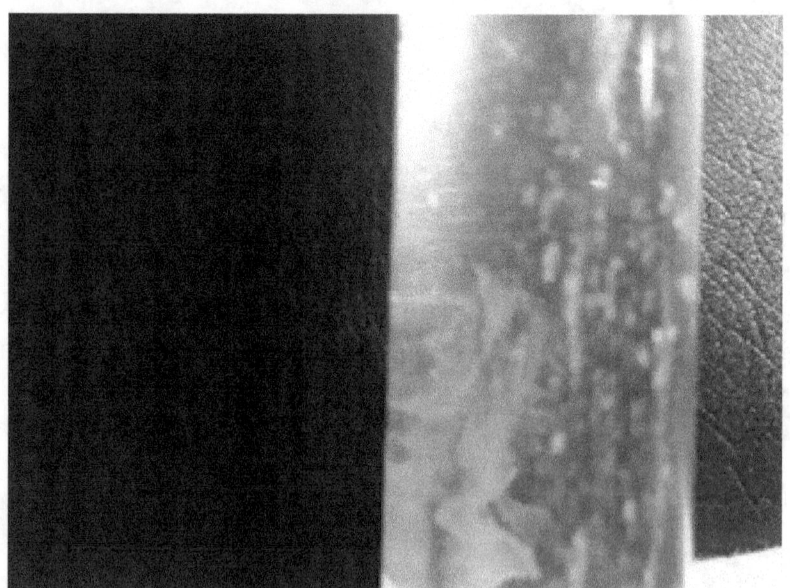

Not liking the looks of that.

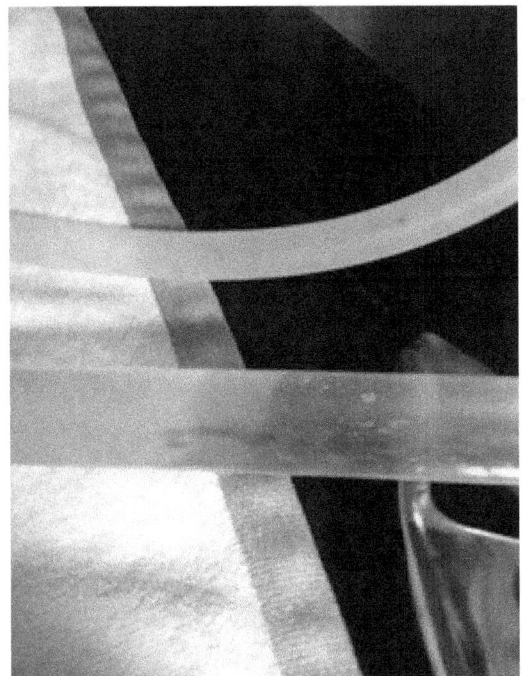

Goodbye little scorpion with hook thing.

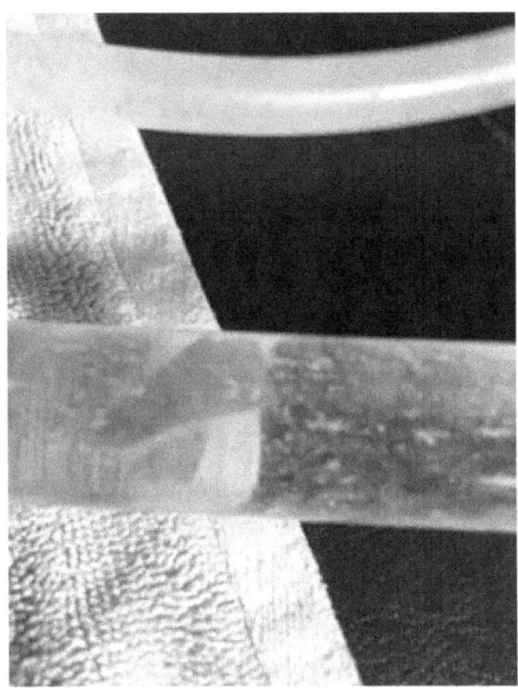

Another pink adolescent fluke. Yawn! So many!

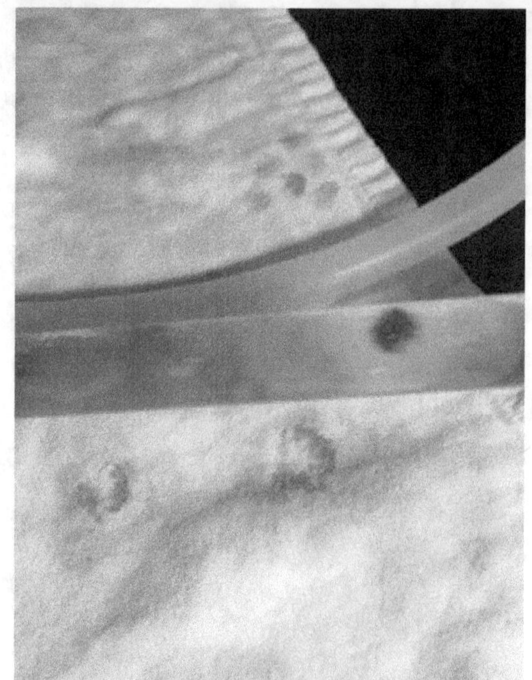

Goo with round floaty ball.

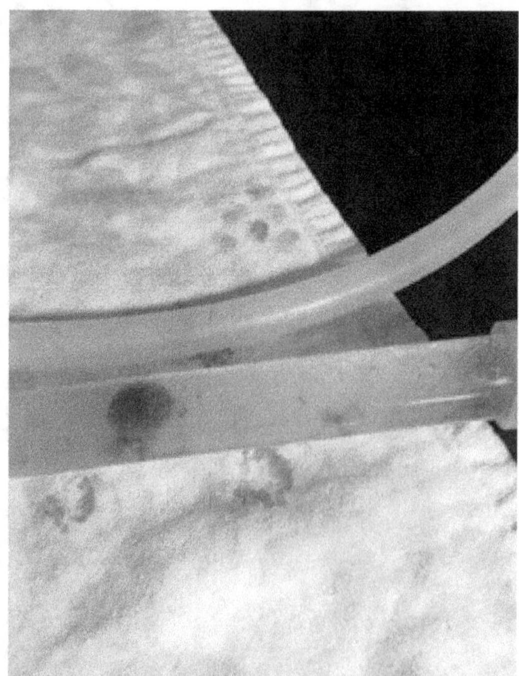

Similar perfectly-formed floaty thing, oval dinosaur egg,
with two legs.

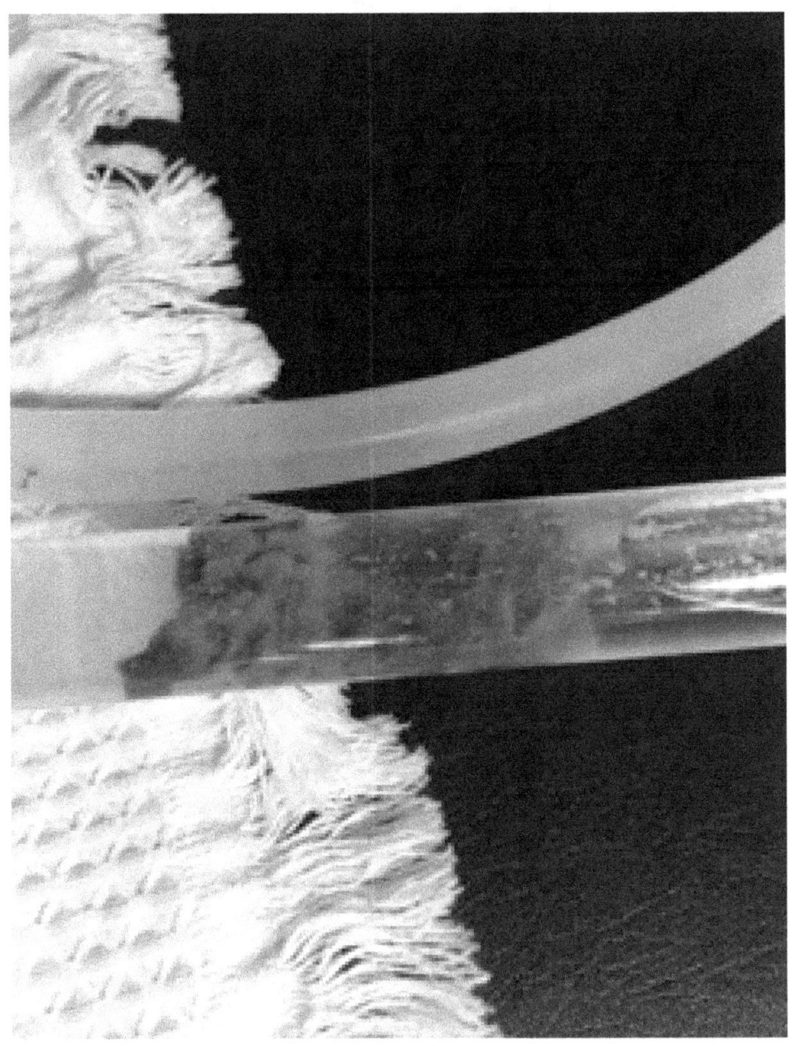

Two gooey balls that look like creepy nests. On right side, that's either an eyeball socket or an opened barnacle pod.

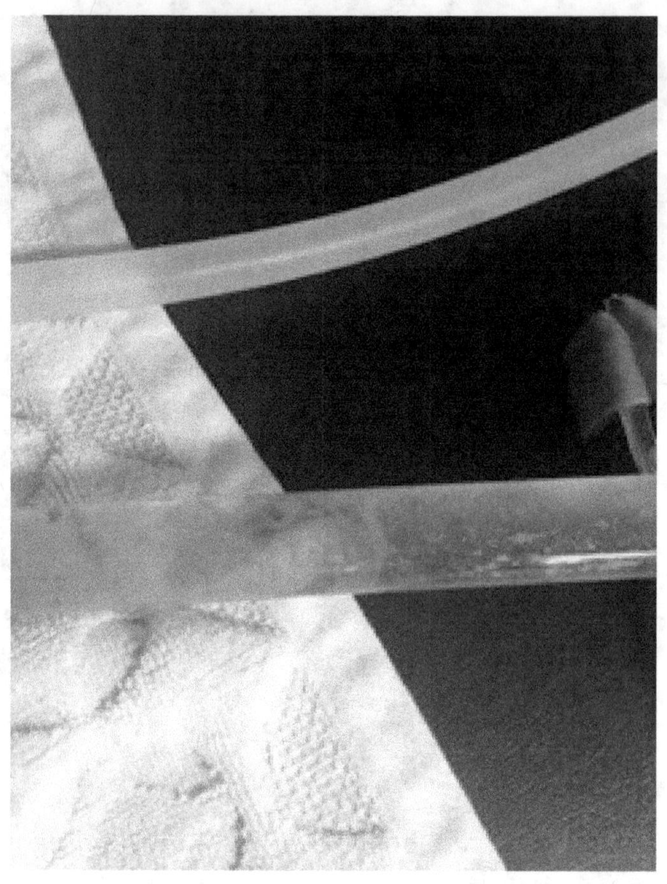

This one is my favorite photo. It's a shrimp-like worm with a BLOW HOLE in the top of its little mucus shell. Here's the thing: I have 140 photos. I'll post them all on my website. Just appreciate that tomorrow I'll spend four or five hours looking at more of these same things coming out from clients, and the next day. You get the sense of it. It's tragic. It's systemic. These things are living in every organ and tissue. I don't know why these aren't showing up in lab reports or medical scans. Human life is precious and people are beautiful. Anybody with the most basic understanding of biology will tell you that beneficial bacteria outnumber the number of individual cells comprising the human's flesh and bone. At the top of the body is a head, your head, with eyes, your eyes, and behind that is a crazy beehive brim-full with other life activity. Within the beehive are a thousand smaller beehives and those have beehives too. I've spent the past 15 years totally avoiding antibiotics for that very reason and consuming probiotic-rich foods way more than the average. My body under my skin is STILL crawling with bug-like things and worms, not just probiotics. I am not exceptional in that capacity, nor are my clients. My colonic office is not responsible for spreading worms. Nashville, Tennessee is not more worm infested than other places in America; not the epicenter. This has been going on for thousands of years and does not matter how long. The worms know all about it and humans don't. This is part of Nature's intelligence. These creatures are not just in our guts. They can travel head to toe. These creatures have been hiding right under our noses. You can leave them as they are and I'm not sure they will harm you all that much. I honestly don't know what to make of it. I also believe these worms influence our blood chemistry and release chemical wastes into our own biological construction. They likely have been designed to measure their total combined affect on everything making up our inner soup. They are beyond smart. I am not aware that they are putting up a fight to stop me from killing them, and it seems like what I have done so far, they accept it as a "system override." The very largest ones are flat and if laid out, could cover the palm of your hand, and most likely reside in the liver. Most of them lay eggs that are between invisible to the size of a poppy seed and a flax seed. Some eggs pass out of the body, but many worm-layers recycle their offspring within. All insects, the kind we do see, help to spread them: gnats, roaches, spiders, flies, ticks, sand fleas, snails, caterpillars. You cannot wash parasite eggs off easily from produce. Their spores are in the dust. We breathe them in. They bring us a simple message. Reality is teeming with life. Our skin does not separate us from IT. There is some correlation of human parasites with the soul, something ELSE that is critical about your being here, something random, while absolutely specific to you. This information is not news to you. You already suspected it. You WANTED to actually know because otherwise it's been confusing. Everything is layers of other things and there's some other message that was once important, but we forgot it. It doesn't matter, because that's part of it. Worms, no worms, there's something funny that is occurring on our planet, a riddle. For some odd reason, a hearty laugh is a significant goal of everything. Even the birds know it and are humbled by a chuckle. The only thing better than waking to the sound of the birds is the sound of people chuckling as we first open our eyes. Other days you will cry. The purpose is to experience every breadth of emotion and to appreciate that your sucking on the bones or the seeds of something else, is okay. Savor every last drop because if you don't, something else will. Nothing can steal anything from you. The most rare thing on the planet is you. You make all the rules. If the rules are changing, you still make the rules. If you are still here, you are probably building some kind of a soul. When you die, somebody will appear and say, "Well done, good and faithful servant." When in another dimension, you awaken to the big irony you sensed was here in this dimension, the elusive hoax made plain. The people who have died ahead of us already know that. It's not a big deal to anybody. Take two giant breaths and let it all go now. If you let it all go now, it won't change much. You are reaching towards the big laughter -- realizing that you are crammed full of parasitic life is part of it. I don't care if you want to kill your own parasitic huddled masses, but if you want to, Angela can help you. I can too. The only reason to kill parasites is because that is your destiny to do so. Where that might take you, I have no clue. Across this particular plane of reality, things tend to die. Every time you move around or boil water, things die. The pyramids in Antarctica serve merely to remind us that it's all temporary. What you know is such an infinitesimal fraction of anything, it can't be all that important. So, take another two breaths and carry on. If you think those two breaths got you ahead, you missed it. Nobody cares if you miss it. They really don't. Pick yourself back up and try again. That's all it is and all the worms on the planet can't stop you. Take two breaths. Nothing can stop you. After you die too, worms will eat out your eyeballs. They will carve little toothpicks from your bones to pick their teeth and the whole rotten thing will sink to the bottom just like the Titanic. Others will barely survive and these will row in little boats towards the light, singing, "Merrily, merrily, merrily, life is but a dream!" A dream. A dream. A dream.

# Chapter 6

# Para•sol

# Protocol + strategies

I've given small bags
of _diatomaceous earth_
to many of my clients.
Some I've asked later—
"Have you been taking it?"
Half have said it's nearly
gone and the other half
say — "I keep forgetting!"

Does it matter to
me whether they take it?
No. I realize that belief
level and motivation will
vary and that's part
of it.

I am not going to launch into any kind of a one-size fits-all thing. Whatever you do, you will want to keep well below the threshhold of feeling <u>overwhelmed</u> or <u>freaked out</u> — always feel like you can <u>joke</u> about it.

Clients have asked me for many years:

Is it BAD?

I always reply:

No, it's fantastic you are here.

It's helpful to catergorize these kinds of things as a <u>learning experience</u>.

Plus, just the fact that you are reading this means that you could be open to new possibilities for some improvement, which previously you hadn't considered. If not, there's plenty of other books about all kinds of things you can read.

I suggest to take this **slowly**. Your inner body is a <u>landscape</u>. Trickles run into small streams, which feed into small creeks, feeding into larger creeks forming into a river leading to a pond, draining into a delta.

The #1 error I see
**ALL THE TIME** is just
like the cartoon cat
getting sucked into the
vacuum hose.

Too **much**, too **fast**.

We've all heard of "the
body cavity."
what that means is that
there is **space** inside.

To begin a parasite cleanse, we would want to begin where FLOW is large and fast. What goes into your mouth enters a relatively large open cavity, which is the digestive tract.



A teaspoon of diatomaceous earth limits parasite cleansing to mainly the intestines.

Adding a little of that to your normal routine is not all that disruptive and more commonly done than most would think. Shop for <u>FOOD GRADE</u> D.E. on the Internet. Some gardening stores sell it too. I am not telling anybody to take D.E., but to <u>consider</u> it and to do your own research. It's fairly ☺ <s>easy</s> to do. If taken with food, it mixes in the stomach, then your food becomes a kind of surprise weapon used against parasites.

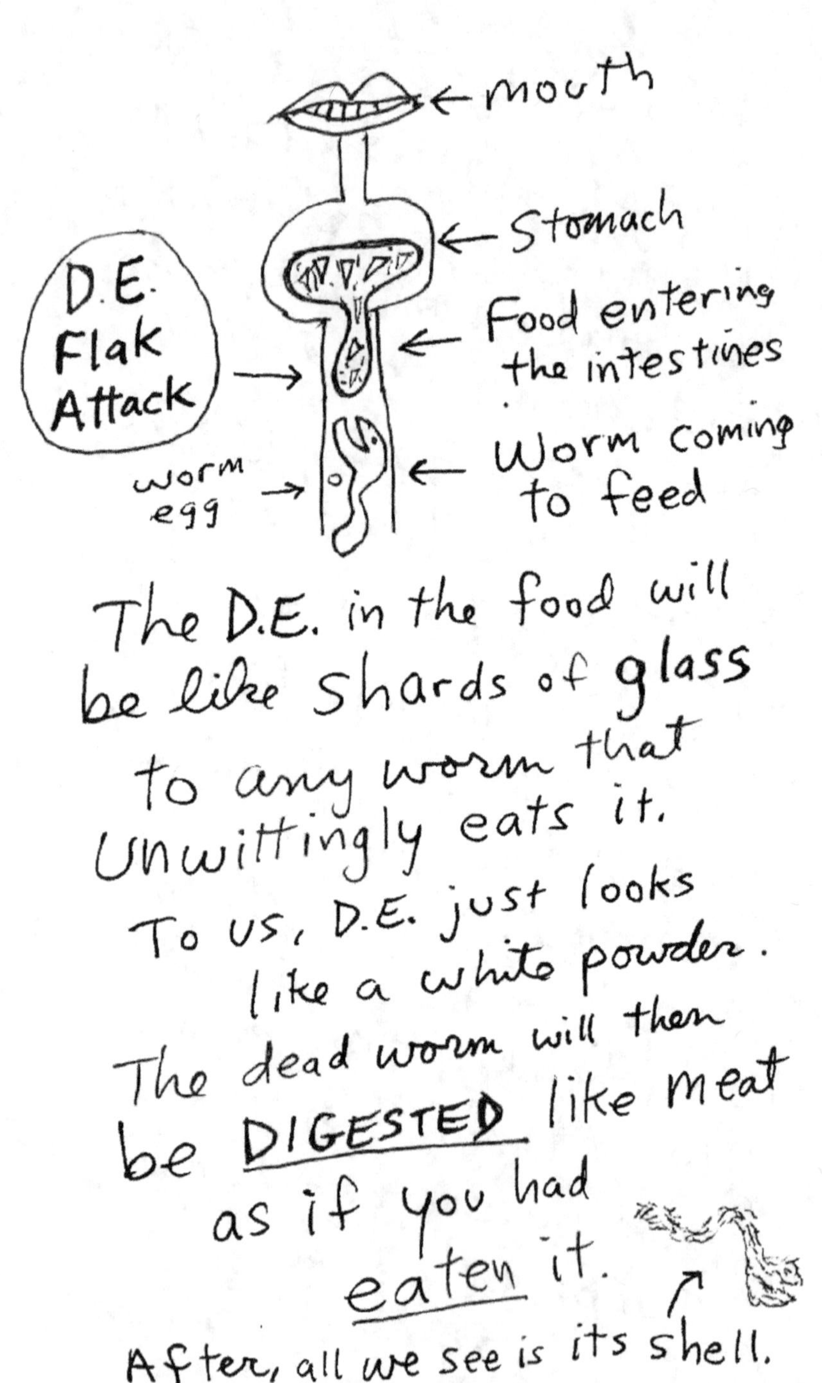


The D.E. in the food will be like shards of **glass** to any worm that unwittingly eats it. To us, D.E. just looks like a white powder. The dead worm will then be <u>**DIGESTED**</u> like meat as if you had <u>eaten</u> it.

After, all we see is its shell.

This is another reason to go **slow**. You don't want to be digesting a lot of dead worms because THAT can make you feel <u>nauseaous</u>. PLUS, parasites might have their own parasites, and if that's a **VIRUS**, you <u>want</u> your natural immunity to kill **it** and so, <u>less is</u> **more**. If all these potential downsides are too scary, and you do <u>nothing</u>, the parasites maybe there in the gut continue to release <u>their</u> <u>waste</u> + maybe lay eggs.....

If you are already ill or have a compromised _immune system_, you could ask your doctor what they suggest you do. Another approach, if you ARE generally sick, is to read articles or books about using creative visualization as a way to TURN UP your _intuition_ and imaginative powers.

From here on, I am going to assume you possess a base line health that will _sustain_ your parasite cleansing efforts.

# #1    One teaspoon daily D.E. with food, in a drink or added to a smoothie.

( D.E. has almost no taste.)

<u>NOTE</u>: Store D.E. away from anything with a strong odor and not near chemicals or cleaning supplies because D.E. is highly absorbant. I keep mine in a glass jar.

With this strategy, you likely won't notice anything different, but any worms in your gut <u>will</u>. Try this in increments: One <u>day</u>. One <u>week</u>. One <u>month</u>. One <u>year</u>.

Also, be careful not to breathe the D.E. powder or get it in your eyes.

NOTE: Your pets can consume D.E. So can children. You can sneak it into their food, but again, I am not telling anybody to do this.

#2 If you have a <u>slow bowel</u>, you will want to speed it up (if your poop could have **dead worms** in it.) Find what will <u>work</u> for you if you haven't already. I myself take one capsule of <u>CAPE ALOE</u> because it works for me.

# #3 Enemas.

Wal-Mart sells a $5 enema bag that lasts for years. I do <u>not</u> recommend <u>FLEET</u> enemas due to additives the manufacturers add.

YouTube offers many instructional videos on it.

If I do an enema, I put in about one cup of warm, filtered water making sure to bleed air out of the hose first. I hold the water while I clean up. INSIDE Then evacuate. Not a lot will come out, but I tend to feel better. Takes 3 minutes, <u>4</u> tops.

#4   The first week, I'd suggest variations of these three things: D.E., a bowel cleanser such a Cape Aloes, and an enema. The next step would be to increase the D.E., from one teaspoon daily to one <u>table</u>spoon daily or one teaspoon 3X daily. You will want to simultaneously protect yourself from viral, bacterial or fungal <u>spin-offs</u> related to dead worms.

I take one capsule of <u>OLIVE LEAF</u> daily. Plus I might take one dropper dosage of <u>colloidal silver</u> every other day, but read the product's description and instructions. I will also take a <u>**yeast cleanse**</u> capsule, or two, every other day which includes tea tree oil, Caprylic acid, Zinc, Vitamin C, grapefruit seed extract and Pau D'Arco.

<u>So far,</u> <u>costs are cheap:</u>
$10 → 2 lbs. Food Grade D.E.
$5 Enema bag    $15 Cape Aloes
$7 - olive leaf
<u>Total monthly cost</u> = $10 or less.

**#5** You are free to <u>stop</u> right there. Try it for a month. Most people will try this for several days, then forget about, come across their bag of D.E. a few months later and say— "Oh yeah! Boy, <u>that</u> was stupid!" Worms!?

**#6** Flax oil and Coconut oil

(refrigerated) ($8–$20) (organic unrefined Raw) ($8–$15)

We will want to begin healing our poor liver versus adding any <u>toxic</u> <u>drag</u> on it. One tablespoon <u>flax + coconut</u> oil each daily. I myself take UDO's brand flax + oil.

#7 One <u>level</u> <u>deeper</u> is to take Sun chlorella tabs. This can help remove "heavy metals" associated with candida, because <u>cleansing</u> ~~yeast~~ will start to unfold. One level deeper is to buy a juicer. I use a $50 Hamilton Beach model from Target. Juicing citrus, especially lemon, with ginger, will help cut <u>mucus</u> in your system. Turmeric + burdock root + celery good for cleansing. One level <u>deeper</u> is consuming more fermented foods like saurkraut, kimchee, kombucha, miso and goat yogurt.

Google: Wild Fermentation ←

<u>NOTE:</u> Less dairy products.
More raw olive oil.
More greens and salads
and seeds.

#8  You've still **not** added
much to do because
you are **BUSY:** You are
taking D.E. and making
sure your poop moves through
daily. You are noticing
that some types of <u>oils</u>
are healthy to support
liver function. You are
reducing MUCUS. Wouldn't
you want to do this
<u>**ANYWAY?**</u>

#9  Now you can do what **Dr. OZ**
suggested — <u>raw garlic</u>. Chew
one medium clove. I myself
cut it with a spoonful of HONEY.

#10   A surprise benefit
is that you will begin to
see things slightly differently.

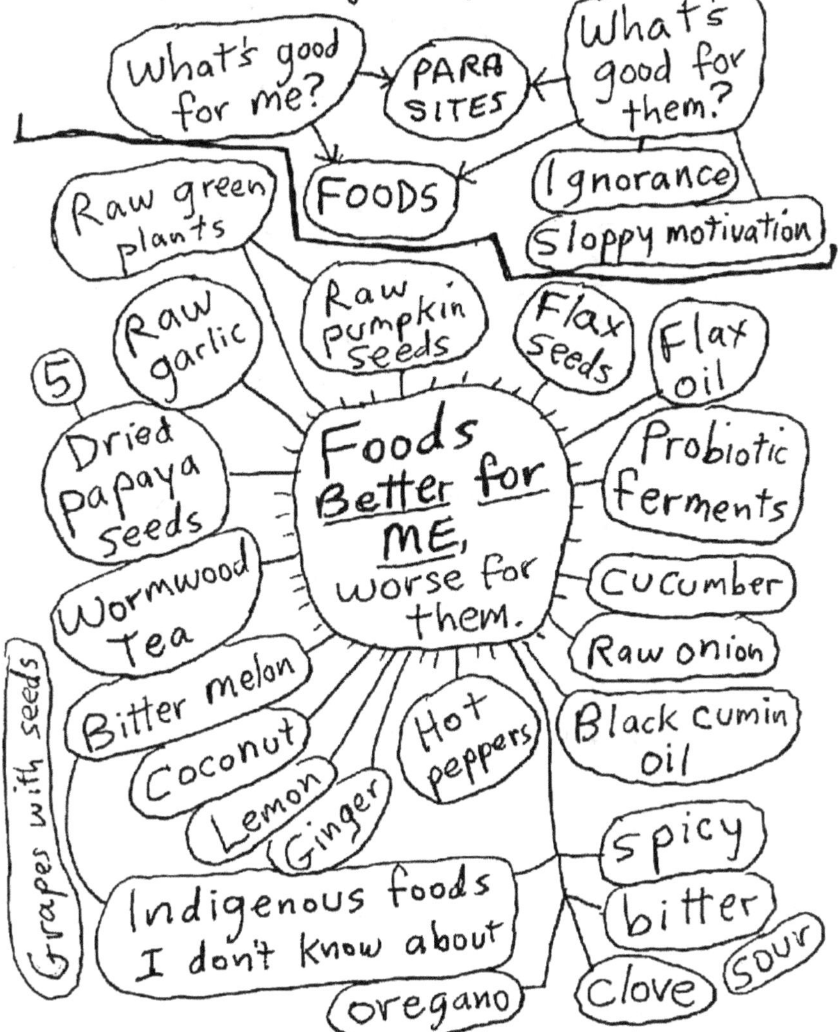

What's good for me?
PARA SITES
What's good for them?
Raw green plants
FOODS
Ignorance
Sloppy motivation
Raw garlic
Raw pumpkin seeds
Flax seeds
Flax oil
5
Dried papaya seeds
Foods Better for ME, worse for them.
Probiotic ferments
Cucumber
Raw onion
Wormwood Tea
Black cumin oil
Grapes with seeds
Bitter melon
Coconut
Lemon
Ginger
Hot peppers
Spicy
bitter
Indigenous foods I don't know about
Clove
Sour
Oregano

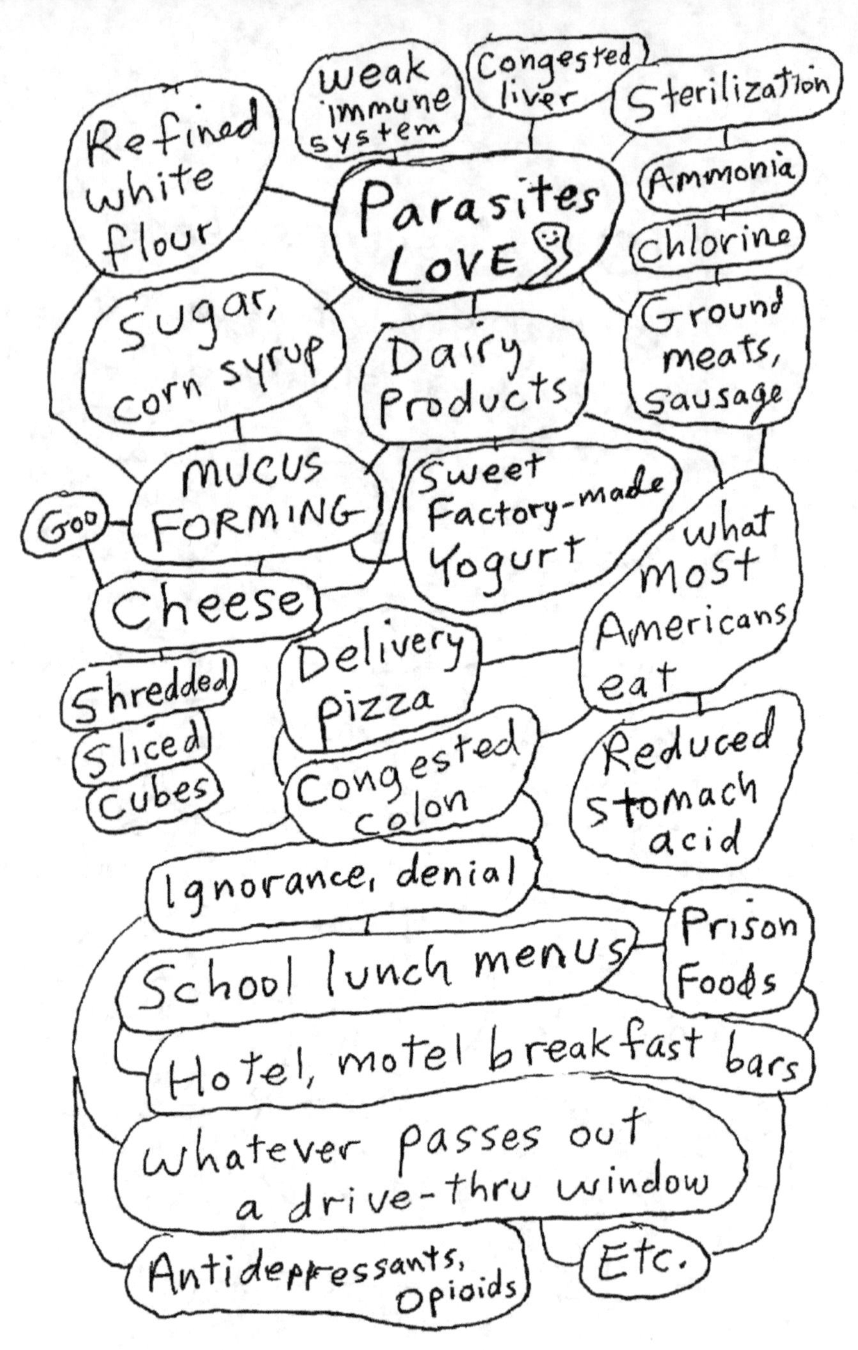

Refined white flour
weak immune system
Congested liver
Sterilization
Parasites Love
Ammonia
chlorine
Sugar, corn syrup
Dairy Products
Ground meats, sausage
Goo
MUCUS FORMING
Sweet Factory-made Yogurt
what most Americans eat
Cheese
Shredded Sliced Cubes
Delivery pizza
Congested colon
Reduced stomach acid
Ignorance, denial
School lunch menus
Prison Foods
Hotel, motel breakfast bars
Whatever passes out a drive-thru window
Antidepressants, opioids
Etc.

# 11   Now that we have the basics down, we are free to do _whatever_ _we want._ Wherever you can break free, relish your FREEDOM.

#12   If you purchase a parasite cleanse KIT in a box, you might be ready for it. We want our lives to be somewhat _Stable_ when we do it. You can't be homeless or starting a new job, or moving, or in the middle of a relational break-up or feel like you could be an emotional wreck for _any_ reason.

It's also wise to clear any **seething hatred** you might feel towards anything or anybody. Because a parasite cleanse can _accentuate_ any and all **emotions** and this part I am **NOT** _joking_ about. We really don't even want to hate our imagined internal parasites. Instead, put yourself in a **happy** place. You can get there **FAST** like snap, snap your fingers. **SHIFT** it, two seconds, snap, breathe. (ok I'm better now.)

#13  You are feeling so OPTIMISTIC now that number thirteen is a lucky number. Notice anywhere in your body that says BLAH! and give it an eviction notice. Tell it: You are **moving out**.

#14 ADVANCED Parasite Cleansing

There are actually lots of experts out there on parasites and cleansing. Awareness regarding the topic is mushrooming and society will understand more tomorrow than today.

One thing about alternative health expertise is celebrity. Celebrity often gets paired with marketing skills. There are not a lot of celebrity <u>colon hygienists</u> partly because their market is mostly localized, so their voices don't get heard at the national level. Celebrity is often built on a base of followers and held together by social media. Glitz is part of it. Glitz generally skims across the surface and returns like a boomerang into the hand of the celebrity who says, "There you have it."

The model that I would propose is that <u>YOU</u> become the expert. Your job then is to form alliances with others who support <u>your</u> journey.



One thing I've observed about Angela is that she writes down her plan, then adjusts on the fly.

She'll say:
- I think I'm taking too much of that.
- I'm going to start taking more of this.
- I need a colonic tomorrow. Whoops, can't make it. I need to rest. Or go to a movie. Or visit with friends.
- I'm sending you a link to a great article or YouTube talk.
- I've changed my mind.
- Going to try something else.
- I wonder what would happen...?
- High five! Give me a hug!
- I'm a little lost right now, but aren't we all?

# #15 <u>Killer Supplements</u>

- **Oxy Powder**
  Believe it or not, oxygen in the digestive tract acts as a kind of poison to parasitic invaders. Take as directed.

- Graviola. As directed.

- **L-Proline/L-Lysine**
  Angela takes five pills the evening or morning before a colonic and swears that it helps to flush out liver flukes.

- **Coenzyme Q-10**
  100 to 250 mg's does a similar thing — kills and flushes worms from the internal organs.

- <u>Liver</u> support formulas.
Just what it says.
- Grafefruit seed extract.
Mild, bitter tonic to kill
candida, a little here,
a little there.
- Barley greens in drinks.
- Shilajit.
Replenishes minerals.
- Pine pollen and Nettles.
- Betaine Hydrochloride. (HCA)
Boosts <u>stomach acidity</u>
which is one line of defense
against parasites.
Over 40? Acidity declines
with age. <u>Pot smokers</u>
will lose acidity too, which
lowers B-12. |MEAT will digest
better with HCA.|

## ∴ Digestive Enzymes

These can be costly,
so if you are low on dough,
split a bottle with a
friend. What you want
is a product high in <u>PROTEASE</u>.
Enzymedica brand makes
one called "Candidase."
This just two enzymes:
Cellulase and Protease.
SOME of your parasites
are not animal, but PLANT.
Protease will rip apart parasitic
protein protection and cellulase
will rip apart cellulose
protection. This also helps
turn up the heat to destroy
anything <u>fungal</u> or <u>Viral</u>.

# Montreal Healthy Girl

Brittany, a Naturopath Health Coach in Canada, provides tons of great information on healing the body <u>long haul</u>. I've never met her or talked to her, but her grasp of things complex and then explaining it in simple terms is amazing. She is an expert on Interstitial Cystitis, a complex malady that represents <u>many</u> ill conditions which overlap and manifest at points of weakness. If anybody can heal IC, they can heal a lot of other things.

Brittany also offers excellent suggestions to reduce **MUCUS**. And, most of what she recommends, she has tried herself.

➳ Asparagus:
One of my clients was eating loads of asparagus as part of a special training diet. Her colonic was full of wormy parasites, along with the fiber of undigested asparagus. I don't know a thing about it other than that. Worms don't appear to like it in bulk.

# Herbal Combinations

Wormwood, black walnut,
green walnut, clove, quassia
and male fern root
are basic to various combos.
I take one or two capsules
of one made by Kroeger
Herb. It's a butt kicker
against worms and I feel
zero side-effects or
die-off issues. These
are made as powders, teas,
tinctures. There is a
wide variety of brands,
prices, mixes, and
endorsements. Go slow,
try them, experiment.

## Bentonite Clay

One major issue is nausea. And even depression. Certainly – gloominess. Here's why:

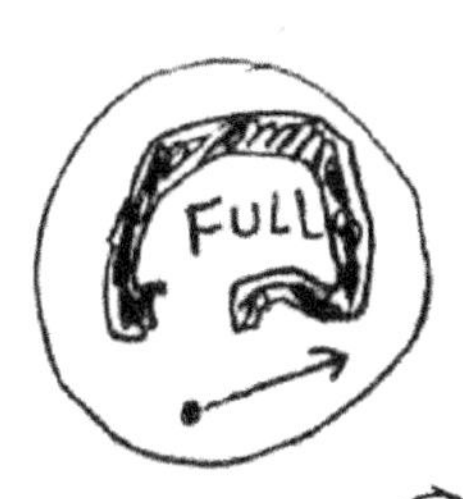


① A slow, congested colon.

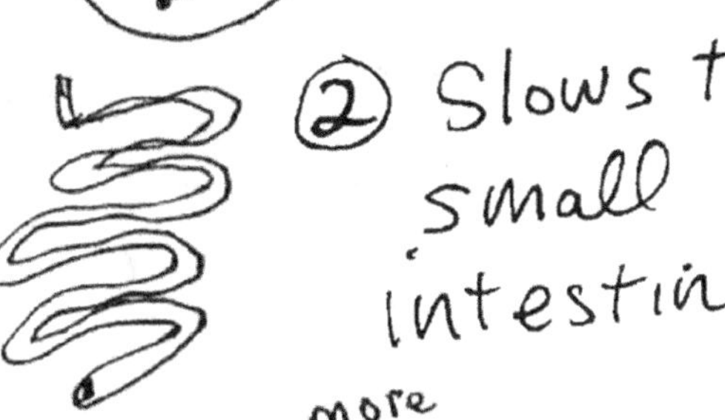

② Slows the small intestine.

③ Causing more DEAD parasites to be digested and absorbed into the blood.

Dead parasites
+
their WASTES

can be engulfed in bentonite clay, their toxic substances absorbed into the clay, preventing their absorption into the human's blood.

Mix food grade clay into water and drink it. Read label.

Even if your colon is not backed up, dead parasites can trigger nausea. ALSO, take a colon cleanser like Cape Aloes to speed transit time. OUT!

CLAY

oh my darling—
Turpentine! ♪♫

I will be adding links to where you can source some of this stuff on my website. **DO NOT** take commercial-grade turpentine you'd buy at the hardware. **SIX** tablespoons could **Kill YOU**. Half a tablespoon (or one teaspoon) will kill worms, but not you. This is distilled pine sap. Too much of **ANY** of these parasite-killing products have diminishing returns, just to be aware.

Not beware. **Be aware.**

My daughter took one
whole tablespoon of food
grade turpentine' and reported
that she could feel it
spreading down her arms,
legs and into her brain.
One _table_spoon is double
what a person might take.
The first time I tried it,
I mixed one _tea_spoon
with one tablespoon of honey.
Some people suggest drizzling
it over 3 sugar cubes. It
doesn't matter — the turpentine
is going to FLY across
your body within
seconds.

What's special about
turpentine is that it penetrates
the many nooks & crannies
under your skin where all
the other parasite cleansers
have CHASED them.
Where? Inside internal
organs, behind eyeballs,
deep in the sinuses, in and
around joints, under the
skull and between skin
and muscle. The first night
after I tried turpentine, I
could feel little wiggles
in places I'd never felt
little wiggles before:
feet, thighs, face,
arms, chest, hips.

I don't take it personally.
I trust I have not lost
my mind. Whatever these
things are, they do _not_
_like_ turpentine. It would
be the same if you drizzed
turpentine over a worm on
the sidewalk — it's gonna
start wiggling more.
        What I do now is to
put a few drops of oregano
oil _directly over_ that spot.
Oregano is more potent
than turpentine. Use
sparingly. It stinks. It burns.
Don't touch it to sensitive
spots like arm pits, eyes,
lips, or the groin.

If the oregano does touch any of those places, you can dilute it with coconut or olive oil. Google what to do if you get it in your eye, just _don't_ get it in your eye! Wash your hands after.

Another _application_ that I apply to wiggles is clove oil. It has the same cautions as oregano oil. I never mix my oils with others when applied to the skin because they are volital.

As effective as turpentine is, it will not wipe out 100% of your internal parasites with one dose.

I've been taking one teaspoon of turpentine with honey once a week for six weeks. I also will rub it on my legs twice a week. It repels chiggers and mosquitoes. I believe a parent could drip a few drops into their hands, rub them together and apply it in the same way as bug repellant for children, but don't quote me on that. Parents seem generally willing to give _medicines_ liberally to their children and this is not much different.

I accept no liability if a parent gets turpentine into their child's eyes or spills it onto clothes. Be careful.

How long will I continue taking turpentine? I have no idea. I am taking all of this one day at a time.

## Medicines

Certainly there are medications created to kill worms. If a med could wipe out 100% of your worms in one day, my belief is that the <u>die-off</u> <u>burden</u> would kill the patient. Or at least send them to bed immobilized.

One of my clients was
on a parasite-killing drug.
He said the pill was outrageously
expensive so he bought his
from Canada, prescribed
by his M.D.  The dosage was
a daily treatment across
six months. He felt
better, but constipation was
a side-effect, hence his
coming to see me. I _don't_
want side-effects. I
take a more indigenous
cultural approach:
utilize Mother Nature
as best we can because
she is our mother.

# Colonics*

While doing all this stuff, some days I feel perfectly fine, normal. I usually poop 3X per day. If I give myself a colonic, which I am doing now three or five days per week, I am absolutely, unequivocally SHOCKED by what exits my body in the colonic water. I will see a whole concoction of wormy things, MUCUS, and foul clouds coming out effortlessly. Usually between 20 to 30 worms ranging in size between macaroni and thumb-size.

I rarely will notice anything weird in the toilet following a bowel movement. It's like two opposite parallel universes. How can I explain it? Not much of what I have written here can I explain. Some days I DO feel nauseous, heavy, toxic. If I do a colonic then, same thing: Instant clouds of little things coming out which belong in the zoo.
Then, I feel 180° turn better.

I'm going to end this story now.

As far as alcoholic beverages _during a period_ of _parasite cleansing_, it's gonna be a long journey. Drink alcohol if it normally contributes to your pleasure. But no more than **two** drinks. Otherwise you are in a danger zone. Life threatening. Or _worst hangover ever_.

It happened to me. Once. Three beers. Never again. See, that's what I've been saying. Therapists and healers have got to try these things _themselves._

Have fun!

# Why BoTOX works:

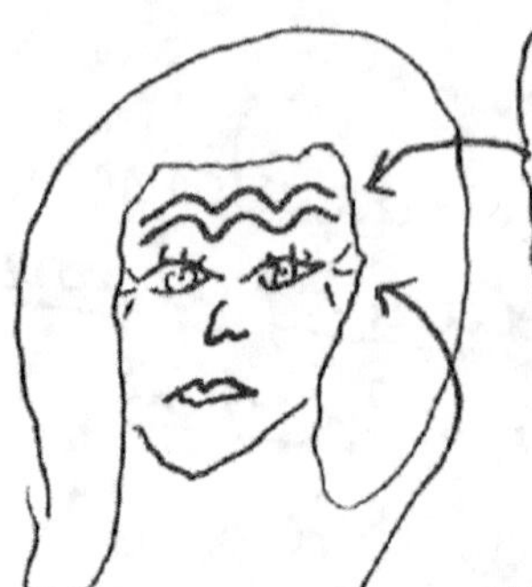




Botox will
paralyze those
worms.

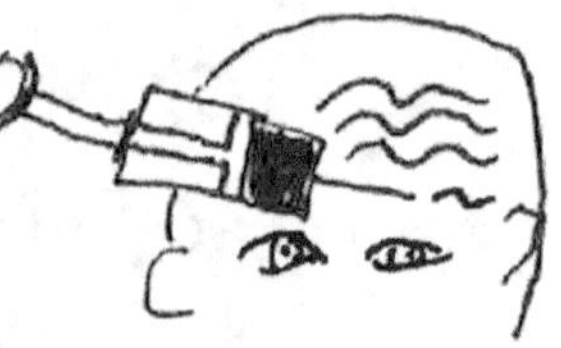

---

# What makes people smile:

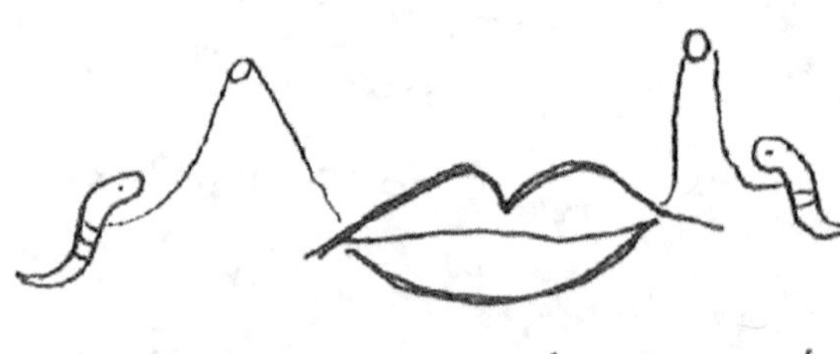


When somebody asks, "Do you
want some candy?" the worms
pull down on the ropes.
The ENTIRE body works this same
way.

We are friends now.
I hope you will consider me to be an ally.

Angela says that she is willing to consult over the phone, while I can vouch for the fact that everybody is BUSY, including her. I told her that if anybody calls her in a panic, to hang up the phone. Given this material has sunk in, anyone who has read it has a full month to do almost nothing except to jot down a strategy outline, do more research and remain calm.

At the top of your strategy will be:



Be specific. If you see yourself wearing shoes, put buckles on your shoes. Imagine in color. Add more color. Add sound: Music, birds chirping, friends laughing. It's less like you just won the lottery, more like you wake up in your bed realizing today is a holiday. Angela is not medically trained and will not diagnose, treat nor prescribe.

If you draw Angela, or me, or anybody else into your circle of support, it is mainly for reassurance that you are on the right track, to avoid pitfalls anybody might unwittingly fall into, trigger new ideas or offer encouragement.

I'll post updates on my <u>website</u>: www.colonic expert.com.

The recommendation for eating <u>papaya seeds</u> is to dry them out, five seeds, ten max, to one tablespoon honey. I sometimes soak one tablespoon of <u>flax seeds</u> overnight in one tsp. (teaspoon) turpentine, chew it in the morning.

If you need more help and are unable to reach me, it's possible that I've left the house and have gone hitchhiking around the country. I may have slept in too, but if you do see me out there with my thumb out, I'd be most grateful for a lift.

In the meantime, see if you can establish contact with a competent and loving colon hygienist near your own neighborhood. If nothing else, it's all about <u>the love</u>.

# Other books I've written:

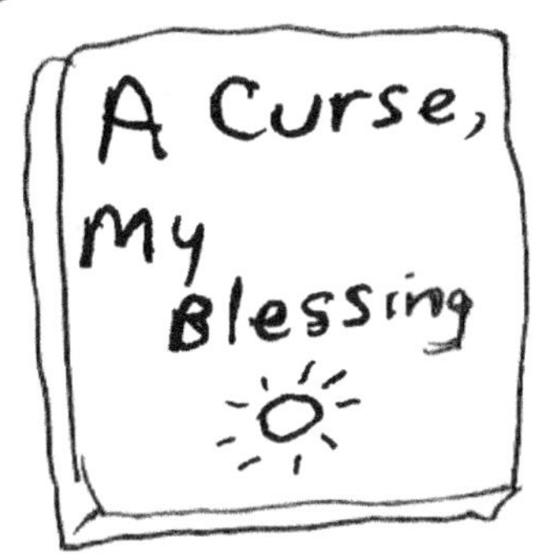


Autobiographic account of my attempts to make sense of evangelical Christianity.

Oh— please either get the new printed version or the digital.

Inside Poop

Self-published in 2006, it's become a niche classic covering the topic of colon hygiene.

The follow-up to Inside Poop. "I couldn't stop laughing."
Joel Salatin

The Conspiracy Theory Diet

The exquisite Donald Trump Down Through HISTORY

The historical backdrop behind how Evangelicals & white supremacists came to support Donald Trump.

www.ingramcontent.com/pod-product-compliance
Lightning Source LLC
Chambersburg PA
CBHW071208240726

48654CB00009B/689